WITHDRAWN

WITHDRAWN

Beautify Bit By Bit

Grow It!

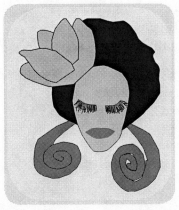

How to Grow
Afro-textured Hair to Maximum Lengths
in the Shortest Time

Chicoro

Beautify Bit by Bit—Grow It! How to Grow Afro-Textured Hair to Maximum Lengths in the Shortest Time by Chicoro

Copyright © 2009 by Chicoro

All rights reserved. No part of this book may be reproduced by any means in any form, photocopied, recorded, electronic or otherwise without the written permission from the publisher except for brief quotations in a review.

ISBN 978-0-9820689-0-8
Library of Congress Control Number 2008908366

Printed in the United States of America

10 9 8 7 6 5 4 3 2 1

Published by ChicoroGYA Publishing
Web site: BeautifyBitByBitGi.com
E-mail: chicoro@beautifybitbybitgi.com

Photographs by Mark Oehler, www.mark-oehler.com
Hair Jewelry Designed by Chicoro and created by Candyce Lyman
Cover Design by BookCoverExpress.com
Interior Design & Typesetting by Jill Ronsley, SunEditWrite.com

Disclaimer

The reader should use their own judgment in utilizing the information in this book. The author and publisher are not professional hair care providers, beauticians, dermatologists, hairstylists or cosmetologists. The reader should seek advice from professionals as needed.

The author's advice and information are based upon years of experience in trying to find a way to attain healthy, thick, long Afro-textured hair. This experience includes research done through studying books, taking classes and working with her own hair and that of other people.

This book is for educational and entertainment purposes. The publisher and author shall have neither responsibility nor liability to any person or entity with respect to any loss or damage alleged to be caused directly or indirectly by the advice or information contained herein.

Dedication

To my precious, wonderful father, who always believed in
my beauty, my gifts, and me. Even today, your advice,
guidance and direction reverberate in my ears.
Daddy, you always said I could do it! I hope that you are proud.
I miss you, but I know that no matter what,
you will always be with me, as you promised.

Contents

Acknowledgments   1

How to Use This Book   3

PART I   **My Story**   5

Chapter 1   Beginning the Journey   7

Chapter 2   The Last Straw   9

Chapter 3   A Ray of Hope   11

Chapter 4   The Discovery   13

PART II   **The Grow It Process**   15

Chapter 5   The Grow It Process Defined   17

Chapter 6   The Science Behind the Grow It Process   19

Chapter 7   The Sole Goal of the Grow It Process   21

Chapter 8   Preserving Your "Dead Ends"   24

PART III   **Grow It Step by Step**   27

Chapter 9   Step 1: All About Detangling   29

Chapter 10   Step 2: All About Cleansing   39

Chapter 11   Step 3: All About Conditioning   46

Chapter 12   Step 4: All About Moisturizing   54

Chapter 13   Step 5: All About Protecting   69

Chapter 14   Step 6: All About Growing   81

Chapter 15   Building Healthier, Longer Hair   100

References   105

Acknowledgments

A big hug and kiss to the four cornerstones who have anchored my life since the day I was born: Christine, Audrey, Janice and Virginia. Your quiet strength, wisdom, insight and support are nothing short of amazing.

To Memo, my favorite photographer and biggest supporter, I love you.

A giant thank-you to my muses, Caroline C. and Miles M. It was Caroline who ever so gently suggested that I write down on paper what I have been sharing with others for years. It was Miles who got me through those blocked walls with an ever-ready encouraging word and endless suggestions.

How to Use This Book

The focus of this book is on how to enhance the growth of your hair and how to capture and retain the growth that you have today. The information is not new, and it is not unbiased or objective. It is my slanted opinion, arising from my view of the hair world. I have based my opinion on research, observation and experience. I have placed my own stamp on this information, to help you Grow It!

This is the first book to focus solely upon growing healthy, longer, natural Afro-textured hair. Wow, that's a mouthful! This book will show you different methods of retaining the length of the hair that grows out of your head.

Certain techniques that are part of the Grow It Process, such as combing the hair with conditioner in it, may not be suitable for relaxed Afro-textured hair, since the strands of relaxed hair can be more fragile than those of natural hair due to the chemical straightening process. I used the entire process successfully while my hair was relaxed, but you will have to be the one to determine which techniques work for you.

This book is intended to be used by those who have relatively healthy hair with no medical hair issues or conditions. The Grow It Process can fit into any and every hair care regimen and routine, including yours. It is not dependent on any ingredient, product or product line. This process is a tool to help you reach your goals and avoid doing those things that get in the way of your goals.

Let your imagination run wild. Use this book to celebrate and support you on your hair-growing journey. Just start with what is on your head. Jump in! Release your preoccupation with perfection. Don't worry about doing things perfectly, ladies. There is no such thing as perfection. Take some risks with your hair, even if at the beginning your risky behavior happens only in front of your bathroom mirror with the door locked. Remember, at any stage you can go back to your usual way of doing things.

In the realm of growing Afro-textured hair, I think I have some tips for you. Come on, let's go! You can have healthier, longer hair. It just takes some faith, knowledge, and a little patience and persistence.

PART I

My Story

Embrace and accept your hair
for what it is today.
Only then can you
discover, cultivate and reveal
its true and priceless beauty tomorrow.

CHAPTER 1

Beginning the Journey

Tyrone, the hair designer, was talking with my mother about me. "You can see through her hair. It's thin and dry," he stated in an impatient, matter-of-fact tone. He was pulling and tugging my hair away from my head, looking at it with distaste. The cutting shears shimmered in his right hand, poised and ready to descend hungrily into my damaged hair. Feeling powerless, with a tearful nod I allowed him to plunge those gleaming, merciless shears into my hair, full force. Tyrone was the expert. He would do what was best for me. Right?

When I entered the shop, I had ponytails that hung to mid-back. After the cut, my hair was layered and it barely fell upon my shoulders. To make matters worse, as I was walking out, Tyrone's fellow stylist looked directly at me and commented to the customer in her chair, "Tyrone didn't have to cut all that child's hair like that."

The health of my hair went downhill from there, and my self-esteem seemed to plummet right along with it. The truth of the matter is that even before I set foot in the hair shop, poor care had damaged my hair. The state of my hair was not Tyrone's fault. It was mine.

My experience that day set me on two pivotal journeys. The first journey was to learn how to become confident enough never to give my personal power away to anyone again. I'd given my power away because I believed the stylist to be the expert. I'd put the fate of my hair into his hands. In other words, I placed accountability and re-sponsibility for myself on someone else, the stylist.

No one can take away your power unless you allow it to hap-pen. Ultimately, you are responsible and accountable for what you allow into your life and what you allow to flow out of your life. It is you who will reap the benefits of your choices, as well as the consequences of those choices. You are accountable for the decisions you make and the actions you take in your life.

The second journey that I began that day was directly related to hair: I was determined to uncover a repeatable, do-able pro-cess for growing long hair. In my case, I was determined to find out how to gain back the length that I had allowed the stylist to take away from me. My own ignorance, my lack of knowledge about my hair, was the main culprit in the demise of its health. It would be knowledge that would turn the situation around.

CHAPTER 2

The Last Straw

*A*ll through high school, I asked every female with long hair, no matter what her ethnicity was, how she attained its length. My famous question was, "How do you grow your hair long?" Even though most girls gave me an answer, none of them really had a clue. They were just as unconscious about how to get there as I was.

Then I heard that a relaxer made hair grow longer. In my senior year in high school, after the school pictures were taken, I decided to get one, too. I didn't like my relaxer, and I started transitioning out of it the day after I first used it. "Transitioning" is simply making a decision not to place any more chemical relaxer products in the hair.

From high school to college, my hair hovered around my collarbone. Sometimes, it would drop to approximately armpit length. Always, it was dry, brittle and roughened with split ends. Through high school and continuing well past college, my long hair was only a memory.

In university, I started growing out my relaxer, which means that I didn't receive any chemical touch-ups on my newly grown roots. I wanted to be free from the relaxer, literally and figuratively. I had found out about curl moisturizer during my last year in high school, and I kept my partly relaxed, partly natural hair saturated with the glycerin-based product.

One day, I was sitting in class at the university. My hair was styled in several thick braids, each one fastened with a coated rubber band. At the end of each braid, below the rubber band, hung an inch or two of loose, unbraided hair. As I sat listening to the lecture, I absent-mindedly pulled and tugged on the loose hair at the end of one of my braids. It was rough to the touch and dull, with a gray cast on the ends. I remember turning my nose up in disgust at my own hair, just as Tyrone had done years before. (Much later, I would learn that this dull cast had a name. It is called weathering.)

Suddenly, the tension of my tugging disappeared. For a split-second, I was confused because I couldn't feel the hair between my fingers anymore. Then I realized that the entire loosened section of my braid, the part that had been hanging just below the coated rubber band, was now resting between my two fingers, free from the braid. Two inches of hair had just broken off! The hair lay in the palm of my hand, lifeless, brittle and crunchy.

I was so ashamed and embarrassed! I held the straw-like hair hidden in my hand until the class was over. I made sure to find a covered trashcan before I felt comfortable enough to release the crunchy, dead hair. I didn't want anyone to see that I knew so little about my own hair that I couldn't even keep it on my head. This was the last straw! I began my search for an answer in earnest.

CHAPTER 3

A Ray of Hope

I read books and articles on how to grow hair. Most of the information was product-centered, which means that it was geared to support the buying and use of a specific product or a full line of products. Some of the information was helpful, but most was just a repeat of what I already knew.

What I knew at the time was very little, and it was not helping me make a lot of progress in getting my hair healthy. Some of the information I found was downright disastrous for my hair. Therefore, I became skeptical about any products or books that claimed to help grow hair.

One day, while flipping through a magazine geared to African-American women, I saw an advertisement for a new line of hair care products. The fashion model in the ad claimed that the products were her own formulation, and that she had grown her hair using them. What caught my eye was the offer of a free booklet on hair care. I called the number and ordered my booklet.

In this booklet, for the first time ever, I saw an African-American woman with relaxed, healthy, waist-length hair. She was sharing her "secrets." From her, I learned about increasing the frequency of washing my hair, and about styling the hair to protect it. She suggested that hair be washed at least one time per week.

Prior to coming across her information, I would wash my hair every other week or only two times per month. Because of her information, I increased the frequency of washing my hair to one time per week.

I wasn't a big fan of her advice on trimming, though. (Later on, I realized that my frequent trimming with no specific goal in mind—as advocated not just by this model but in other articles and books I had read—was a big part of why my hair had stayed short.) But the important thing was that she made things seem so simple. She said that growing hair to great lengths was easy.

I had finally found someone who validated what I'd believed all along: it was possible to grow long, healthy Afro-textured hair. By then, I was able to grow my hair down my back, but it became split, dry, thin, and still gray and brittle at the ends. It never looked silky when I straightened it. I thought that if I applied heat to my hair, it would get straighter. I would not learn until years later that the healthier the hair, the less heat you have to apply to get your hair to shine and gleam.

CHAPTER 4

The Discovery

Sometime after college and well into my career, I got a job in Mexico. This was the good news. The bad news was that I was transitioning out of a second permanent relaxer, and I knew that I would not seek out the services of a beautician in Mexico to get touch-ups. Still, I was not going to pass up a dream job and the opportunity of a lifetime just because of my hair.

I tried to keep my mixture of partially natural, partially permanently relaxed hair for as long as I could. Unfortunately, when at least a year had passed since my last touch-up, my relaxed hair started to break. I decided to cut it, so that I would be left with only natural hair. After the cut, the length was back to my collarbone. The ends were free of split ends, free of knots and soft to the touch, but once it started to grow past my shoulders, the ends got rough again.

Now I discovered that the ends of my hair needed special care. They needed to be kept moist, and the moisture needed to be locked into the hair. I experimented with different ways to accomplish this. Over time, I made discoveries, and I refined what I learned. This evolved into the Grow It Process.

The Grow It Process is a model. A model is the way one views the world. A model allows you to sift and sort the abundance of data that comes to you every day, so that it can fit into your belief system and world view. This simply means that any established model enables you to peruse information as it comes in and quickly determine what fits into your current belief system. Most of us keep what matches our beliefs and discard what does not.

Be careful about what you deem to be true and untrue. Be meticulous and conscious about how you build your model. Once it is in your head, it is difficult to get rid of or modify. The worst and most detrimental model pertaining to hair is the belief that Afro-textured hair cannot grow long. If this is the model you have in your mind, at least you have suspended that belief for a moment. Otherwise, you wouldn't be reading this sentence.

What is the Grow It Process?

PART II

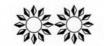

The Grow It
Process

*A single bead of liquid, dropped into a
large body of water, makes concentric
circles that have an impact farther
than one could imagine.
Tiny adjustments, one at a time,
can do wonders for your hair.
Pursue your hair goals not as superficial
endeavors. They may lead you to places
that you have only dreamed of.*

CHAPTER 5

The Grow It Process Defined

There are six steps to the Grow It Process. They are defined below:

1. Detangle your hair prior to washing it. Detangling is a two-part process. First you detangle the hair when it is dry; then when it is wet. Begin with just your fingers.

2. Cleanse your hair frequently. One time per week is a good starting point. Some may prefer to wash more frequently. Others may prefer to wash less frequently. Styles, products and personal preferences will dictate the frequency of washing. Dirty hair, hair burdened with product, is more prone to breaking than clean hair.

3. Condition your hair intelligently. Just because a bottle says "conditioner" doesn't mean that it is what you need at this point. The needs of your hair should dictate your selection and use of conditioner.

4. Moisturize your hair. This always involves some water-based or liquid product. Moisturizing can be as simple as just using water or as complex as making your own product.

5. Protect your hair. This allows you to shield your priceless hair from anything that might damage it. It is possible to wear your hair completely loosened and still protect it.

6. Grow your hair. This seems to be something over which you have no control. You do, though! I will show you a trimming technique that helps you to have thick, full, even ends faster than you can with ordinary trimming techniques. I call it the Goal Point method. It is a method of trimming that affects your state of mind more than the physical growth of your hair.

These steps can be accomplished with any ingredient or product of your choice and any regimen of your choice. Not every product works for every head of hair. Discovering your products of choice is something that you must do for yourself by trial and error. No one can do it for you. The Grow It Process can help to reduce your learning curve.

The difference with the Grow It Process is that it's a process you can easily follow. It is not product-focused, which means that it has not been designed to work or be used only with specific products. This model provides a base. Once you have understood and internalized the Grow It Process, you can modify it to fit your lifestyle. You can use it in conjunction with the products that work for you in your current routine, or with products that you have yet to discover on your journey.

CHAPTER 6

The Science Behind the Grow It Process

There is science behind the Grow It Process. I didn't discover the science until long after I had implemented the process, and my hair had been healthy for years.

Did you notice that I used the word "discover," and not "invent"? A good model is based on natural laws. Natural laws are built on truths that can only be discovered, not invented. The science behind the Grow It Process is really the science of hair. This science is important to know and understand.

When you understand a process, it becomes meaningful for you. You can use it as a model to analyze your own situation and apply what works for you. You will develop insight so that you can determine what action within your hair care regimen may need to be modified, eliminated, increased or decreased. You will be able to determine whether the issue or barrier that keeps you from reaching your goal is process-specific, product-specific, or whether it arises from another cause.

Without knowledge, you will forever be guessing about what you should do for your hair.

With knowledge, you can determine what best suits your particular circumstances. Knowledge of the science of hair that is meaningful and applicable to your lifestyle will allow you to exercise discernment in what you do to your hair and what products you select.

No longer must you hungrily wait by the seashore in hopes that someone will toss you a fish, which you gulp down only to be left dissatisfied and hungry. The fish can be likened to a tidbit of information about a magic product, which always turns out not to be so magical after all. With knowledge, you develop skill. Skill allows you to stand confidently upon those same shores and do your own fishing. Knowledge can help make you independent, autonomous and powerful.

With knowledge, the learning curve is smoothed out. You may take less time to find the process that works for you. Your trial-and-error period may be shortened, so that you arrive at a good regimen with products that work for you faster than you ever anticipated. Skill will help you to refine your hair care process, whittling away the junk and noise of useless products and actions that leave your hair just like it was before—or that leave your hair in worse condition, and you with lighter pockets.

Skill will guide you and help you see that there is no miracle product. You will learn that what works for someone else may not work for you. You will also learn that products and techniques that do not work for others may work wonderfully for you. This is the main reason that I do not recommend a specific line of products. I may mention and recommend a few products and an ingredient here and there, though.

It is time to be responsible and accountable for your hair success. It is time to take your hair care into your own hands. Part of that responsibility is discovering what products work best for your hair. No one can give you that knowledge. To be truly successful, you must find it on your own.

CHAPTER 7

The Sole Goal of the Grow It Process

The sole goal of the Grow It Process is to preserve for as long as possible the natural structure of each and every strand of hair currently on your head.

In simple terms, the structure of each hair strand is made up of the outermost layer, called the cuticle (each strand of hair has several cuticle layers); inside them, the cortex; and then the innermost part of the hair strand, the medulla. Some hairs may not have a medulla, but we are focusing on what exists in general. Most strands of hair have a medulla.

This structure, composed of the cuticle, cortex, and medulla, is meant to remain intact and in place for the entire life of each strand of hair that grows out of the scalp. This time frame is approximately three to six years. The structure of each hair, composed of the cuticle, cortex and medulla, is supposed to stay in place for at least that many years.

Just like everything else, hair ages over time. It experiences wear and tear. This is called weathering. The degree of weathering and the speed at which hair becomes weathered are greatly dependent upon what you do to your hair. The speed of weathering is also dependent upon what you don't do to your hair.

Weathering is damage. Weathered hair is damaged hair. Damaged hair is weakened hair. First, the cuticle, the outermost part of the hair strand, begins to break down. Eventually, the entire cuticle may disappear layer by layer until it is completely worn away. This exposes the cortex of the hair, which is very vulnerable. The cortex is protected by the cuticle of the hair; once the cortex is exposed, the hair begins to split.

Most of us notice splits at the ends of our hair, but a split can also occur in the middle of the hair shaft (strand) or even higher, near the roots. Once the hair begins to split, it is likely to break. Split or broken hair has been stripped of its natural cuticle structure.

The focus of a successful and beneficial hair care regimen for any type of hair is to preserve the cuticle, also called the scale structure, of the hair for as long as the hair is attached to the scalp. This will extend the life of the hair strand.

If you are able to maintain or extend the life of the hair strand, it remains on your head for a longer time. The more time the hair is on your head, the more time it has to grow. The more time it has to grow, the more opportunity you have to capture and retain that growth. The more growth you retain, the longer the hair.

It is quite possible to retain length but to have dry, brittle, split, unhealthy-looking long hair. For many years, that was the case with my hair. Therefore, it is not enough just to retain length. The goal is to retain healthy length. The only way to do this is to maintain the structure of the hair strand.

Just as some actions that you take expedite the damage visited upon your hair, you can also take actions that slow down the damage. You can use products that replace, or mimic, the hair structure once it has been damaged or worn away. You can take actions to help the hair appear healthy. The purpose is to avoid any damage to the hair, although that is not always possible.

Let's put it all together. The sole goal of the Grow It Process is to preserve the natural structure of every hair strand for as long as possible. The focus of any hair regimen should be on preserving the cuticle, or scale structure, of the hair for as long as the hair is attached to the scalp. The goal is to retain healthy length.

Hair structure is basically the same across all ethnicities and races. However, the physical characteristics of the hair differ from one ethnic group to another. These differences give rise to different preferences in products and styling methods. The only constant you need to adhere to is to learn and understand the process or model that supports your key goal.

The key goal is for you to preserve the natural structure of your hair. Once you understand and internalize this basic goal, you will have the tools and knowledge to customize your regimen so that it fits your preferences and hair needs. This is the reason that the Grow It Process is not dependent upon a certain ingredient, product, product line or style.

If you truly understand the mechanics of what you need to do to preserve the natural structure of the hair strand, you will be released. You will be free to choose products, regimens and styles most appropriate for your hair and your life. This is the hair equivalent of teaching you to fish for a lifetime, instead of giving you a fish to eat only for today.

CHAPTER 8

Preserving Your "Dead Ends"

With some notable exceptions, experts agree that, technically, hair is dead. Confusion persists, though. How often have you heard someone say, "I need to remove these dead ends"? There is partial truth in this statement.

It is not just the ends of the hair that are dead; the entire strand is dead. What the speaker is usually referring to is the broken, split or generally damaged part of the strand. This is the part of the hair where the structure has been permanently damaged or stripped.

When hair is alive inside the scalp, the keratin in the hair becomes hardened. Keratin is a protein made up of amino acids. The hair beneath the scalp becomes keratinized, which means the protein in the hair becomes hardened. It is then pushed out by the growth continuing to occur in the hair follicle. Once the hair is pushed out of the scalp, it no longer experiences cell division. Cells that are no longer dividing are dead cells. Therefore, the hair strand is made up of dead cells: the cells are no longer dividing, so the hair is dead. That is why I believe that the focus of any hair regimen should be on the preservation of the hair strand. When something is dead, and you want to keep it around, you try to preserve it.

Because the intact structure of the hair is what gives hair its healthy appearance, you want to preserve the state of the hair structure. This means that you want to keep the structure the same as it was when it first poked through the scalp. Reaching the goal of having healthy-looking hair depends upon how well you preserve the scale structure of the hair. If you keep this thought in the back of your mind, it will be easier for you to recognize and understand what processes and techniques you need to incorporate in your hair care regimen. You will see how your daily, weekly and monthly routines either support you or hinder you in your attainment of your goal.

Even though the hair shaft is technically dead because its cells are no longer dividing, we may describe it as healthy. But over time, its properties, such as porosity and flexibility, can change so much that the hair loses its healthy appearance. The ends or the tips of the hair are the parts that are most vulnerable to change and subject to breakage.

Detangling your hair directly with combs and brushes tends to strip the cuticle, or scale structure, of your hair. Once the scale structure has been completely stripped or removed from the hair strand, the hair may split and break. This splitting results in the fragmentation of the cortex, which has been exposed because of the missing cuticle layer.

One function of hair conditioner is to reduce friction on the hair. This reduction of friction helps with the detangling process, lessening the chances of stripping the scale structure. The scale structure of the hair is thus preserved for a longer period of time, which means that you have a longer period before the hair shows signs of wear, or begins to split or fracture at the tip. Therefore, the first step of the Grow It Process is detangling.

PART III

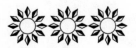

Grow It
Step by Step

Build your process like a pyramid.
Spiral upward until you reach the apex.
Document what you do.
You never know who you will inspire
with the footprints of your journey.

CHAPTER 9

Step 1

All About Detangling

*B*efore you begin to detangle, remember never to try to detangle your hair when you are preoccupied, in a hurry or not in the mood to be patient with your hair. If you do not have time, leave the tangled hair for another day. In detangling your hair, haste truly makes waste.

The most damage can occur when performing the detangling process. When you are detangling your hair, you are placing pressure on your hair from pulling it, stretching it and exposing it to stripping, ripping and tearing from mechanical implements such as brushes and combs. Let's face it, hair tangles and you can either let it dread and matt, cut it out or detangle it. For our purposes, we are trying to gain length on loosened hair. Therefore, the preferred option to reach our goal is to detangle the hair.

No matter when you detangle hair, whether you perceive your hair to be dry or wet, your hair is always vulnerable to damage during this step. This is because unless the atmosphere or environment is totally devoid of or completely lacking moisture in the air, the hair is never really completely dry 100% of the time. Hair that is never completely dry is moistened or wet. Wet hair is weakened hair. Weakened hair is vulnerable to breakage. Why is this? This is because water, or moisture in the air, temporarily breaks certain bonds and linkages of the hair. It is from the connectivity of these bonds and linkages that the hair gains it strength. In other words, when these bonds and linkages are in place, the hair is at its strongest.

Hair is hygroscopic: it readily attracts water from the surrounding air and retains the water in place wherever hydration is needed. This means that you do not have to place water or moisture in your hair in order for it to be wet. In contrast, hair that is porous, which is hair that has lost its ability to hold water, is damaged hair. Hair that is overly porous can be dry and brittle. Porous hair is vulnerable because some aspect of the hair structure is cracked, broken, missing or damaged in some way. Thus, when hair is referred to as being hygroscopic, the assumption is I am discussing healthy hair with its structure intact, as opposed to damaged hair that no longer has its structure in place.

Healthy hair is very strong because of its chemical constituents and its chemical make-up. This includes, but is not limited to, hydrogen bonds, salt links and the arrangement of keratin fibers. When hair is wet, chemical constituents such as the salt links and the hydrogen bonds of the hair, are temporarily broken until the hair is completely dry. The tricky part is that due to the hygroscopic nature of hair, if there is moisture in the air, dry hair can quickly become moist enough and/or wet enough hair to break the bonds and links. Because the breaking of the bonds and links is a chemical reaction, you may not be able to tell whether or not your hair is wet from feeling it or touching it. Therefore, your hair can be wet even when it feels dry to the touch.

This is important because it is the bonds and links in the hair that give it its strength. When the hair is wet, these bonds are temporarily broken until the hair is dried. When these bonds and links are temporarily broken, the hair is in a weaker state. Since most of us can't pull out a moisture kit to measure the moisture in the air and on our hair, it is best to assume that there are always some broken links and bonds in the hair at all times. Therefore, no matter when or where you are, it is always important to handle the hair with care. Never assume that because your hair is dry to the touch that you can be less gentle with it. Your hair is always vulnerable to breakage because it is never completely dry as long as there is moisture in the air. Whether your hair is healthy or damaged, in either state, when it is wet it is weaker.

Always assume that damage can happen to hair during the detangling step because the hair is always potentially wet. Wet hair is more vulnerable to breakage than drier hair because the bonds and linkages that create the strength in the hair are temporarily broken when wet. Thus, it does not matter whether your hair feels dry to the touch or sopping wet. You must always detangle your hair with the utmost of care.

Keep the Hair Dry and Use Your Fingers to Detangle It

If your hair is dry, immobile, brittle or hard because of the use of certain products, such as hair gels or leave-in products, skip the dry detangle step. Just proceed directly to the wet detangle explanation. If you have been wearing very small braids—usually more than ten braids for more than one month, without taking them down—you should also skip the dry detangle method and proceed directly to the wet detangle explanation.

Whether your hair is in a natural or straightened state, it is best to begin the detangling process when the hair is dry. Detangling should be done without wetting the hair, and using only your fingers. We are assuming that the hair is not caked hard, or so greasy and gummy with product that you cannot get your fingers through it. If the tangles and the product build-up are at a minimum, you should be able to begin with the dry detangling method. The reason for dry detangling is for you to determine where your hair is tangled.

Using your fingers, remove all hairpins, clips and adornments from your hair. Use your fingers to section the hair. Try to divide the hair into four sections, perhaps two sections in the back and two in front. If your hair is very tangled, you may be able to section your hair into only two sections, such as two ponytails, one on either side of your head or one on top and one on the bottom. Don't worry about having a straight part between each section. Just section the hair as best you can.

Decide which section of hair you want to focus on, and tie the rest of the hair back out of the way. I like to use a nylon knee-high to tie back the hair on which I am not working. Old nylons and nylon knee-highs do not catch, pull or tear my hair, and they are inexpensive to use. There is no need to cut the nylon knee-high. Just use it as is, like a giant, thick string, and wrap it around your hair.

Now focus on the section of hair that you wish to detangle first. Grip the section at the roots, as if you were about to put it into a ponytail. Gently encircle the sectioned hair with your hand. While still holding onto the hair, move your hand from the roots to the tips of your hair. Try to get all the hair in that section smoothed and going in the same direction. The smoothed and natural direction of the cuticle structure is downward, away from your scalp. You may need to go over the hair with your hands several times to smooth it. It is okay if your hair still has tangles at this point.

Identify any tangles in this section of hair. Do not use a comb. Using your fingers, find a tangle and gently pull away as many hairs as you can from around the tangle, a few at a time, until you reach the very core of the tangle. You will know you are at the core of the tangle when you cannot remove any more hair from it without risk of breaking the hair. Usually, the core tangle will be stuck together because of gummy hair product, dust or a piece of hair that has broken off, wrapped itself around the other hairs and captured them. The broken piece of hair may even have become knotted. Knotted hair is not a function of unhealthy hair. Babies, who have the healthiest hair and perfectly intact cuticle structures, can get knots in their hair, too. Because of its curl pattern, Afro-textured hair, or any curly hair, has the tendency to knot.

Squeeze the core tangle and move it by rubbing it between your fingers. This will loosen the tangle. In general, you do not want to rub your hair together; that is why we try to find the smallest core component of the tangle before rubbing it. Since the core tangle will consist of only a few hairs, rubbing them together at this point is more likely to assist the detangling process than to cause damage. Try to separate the hair from the core tangle, hair by hair. Once you have reached the core tangle, you should not have too many hairs to deal with.

What if you can't remove the core tangle? Pat yourself on the back because you have not ripped through it and broken your precious hair. Pat yourself on the back again because you have reduced the size of the tangle. These are definitely accomplishments. This is progress.

Yes, it takes patience. But wouldn't you rather take an extra few minutes, or even an extra hour, to detangle your hair so that you have minimum breakage and thus retain your hair? Or would you rather rush through the detangling step, tear through your hair, pull out entire curls and have to take months to try to repair the damage?

If you cannot remove the tangle, leave it for now. Comb your fingers through the section of hair one more time. You still may not be able to get your fingers through the section because of some remaining tangles. That is okay, as you will have reduced the amount of hair involved in the tangles. The goal of detangling your dry hair with your fingers is not to remove every single tangle. The goal is to get your hair to the point where it is detangled enough so that you can further section it without creating more tangles or matting the hair. (If your hair is matted when it is dry, proceed directly to the wet detangle discussion.)

Now isolate the detangled section by either twisting it out of the way or pinning it up and away from the hair that is yet to be detangled. Do not leave it loose. You do not want the section to tangle again, or to get mixed up with the hair that is still to be detangled. You do not want to create unnecessary work for yourself.

Repeat this process until you have detangled all your dry, sectioned hair. You should not be using a comb or brush or wetting your hair at this point in the process. Use only your fingers. The goal is to get your hair detangled enough so that you can divide it into distinct sections.

When you have succeeded in detangling your hair, divide it into small sections and braid each section loosely. (If your hair is tangled but it is too short to braid, skip the dry detangle step and proceed to the wet detangle step.)

Wet the Hair and
Use Your Fingers to Further Detangle It

If you have managed to completely detangle the hair while it is dry, meaning you have not placed water in your hair or any other product in your hair to moisten the hair, section it and loosely braid it. Once the hair is braided, it is still a good idea to rinse those braids under water. The hair benefits from being wet or rinsed with water as this will wash some of the dirt, grime or product from the surface of the hair. Although wetting the hair weakens the individual strands, there is strength in numbers because the individual strands are protected within the braid. The hair will benefit from rinsing as this will soften the hair strands. The fact that it is wet and weakened is balanced by the fact that individual hairs are fortified and strengthened because they are grouped in a braid. You will be handling the wet braid with a bulk of hair as opposed to single, wet individual strands.

If you are still detangling you're your hair because you are unable to detangle it without wetting it, you still may need to make one more decision. Before wetting your hair, it is important to determine what you should use to wet it. Sometimes it is appropriate to use just water. At other times, it may be necessary to wet your hair with a water-based conditioner or even some type of oil. The state of your hair should determine what type of liquid you should use. You will have to make this decision yourself.

You may use some or all of the following techniques in your routine.

When to Wet the Hair with Water

When the hair is hardened or matted, it is usually due to product build-up. At these times, you may want to use water to help with the detangling process. In addition to rinsing your head under running water, you can mix two parts B panthenol with twenty parts water, place it in a spray bottle and saturate your hair with it before you take down your hairstyle or braids.

Hardened Hair

If the core tangle is due to your hair being hardened from product build-up, it is best to first wet the hair with water. When the hair is immobilized by gel, hairspray or any other type of product, you want to try to remove the product. The purpose of the water is to rinse as much product from the hair as possible without combing the hair. This should soften the hair so that it becomes supple. Then you will be able to manipulate your hair, moving your fingers through it with minimum resistance and thus less breakage. Section the hair.

At this point, you do not want to use any type of clarifying product, such as clarifying shampoo, vinegar or lemon juice on your hair. If you have too much vinegar or lemon juice in your rinse, or if the commercially prepared clarifying product is too acidic for your hair, it will have the opposite of the desired effect: it will lift the cuticle. Acidic products that lift the cuticles create little, upward-jutting hooks on the cuticle, which make the hair more likely to catch on other hairs that are touching it or near it. Your hair will feel roughened. Your goal now is to smooth out the cuticle of the hair as much as possible, so that you can get it detangled. Since it is hard to gauge what is too acidic for your hair, skip these products for now.

Matted Hair

If the core tangle consists of matted hair, this could be because loose hair that is no longer attached to the scalp has become intertwined with the other hair, or it could be due to product build-up or to a combination of the two factors. Use water to try to soften the matted section of hair. Once the matted section has been moistened, gently try to pull the hairs apart. You may tear some of your hair, but you definitely have to tear apart, separate and remove any hair that is no longer attached to the scalp but may be still intertwined and interspersed amongst the hair you want to retain. Section the hair.

Thin, Fine or Oily Hair

If the core tangle is in thin, fine or naturally oily hair, water is probably the best option to use to continue the detangling process. Section the hair.

Very Short Hair

If the core tangle is in hair that is too short to section, it may be a good idea to wet it with water. Depending upon the nature of the core tangle, you could also use conditioner or oil to moisten the hair to continue detangling it.

When to Wet the Hair with Water-Based Conditioner

If the core tangle in your hair is gummy, this could be due to product build-up from petroleum, wax-based hair grease, or even from natural oils or butters that you have placed in your hair. Conditioner can sometimes dissolve the oils from the core of the tangle, because many of the conditioners available today have surfactants, or cleaning agents, among their ingredients (see Chapter 10: All about Cleansing, for a discussion of surfactants.) Use water-based conditioners, which are thinner in consistency than cholesterol-type conditioners, directly on the hair and on the core tangle. You will still need to work your fingers through the tangle, separating as many hairs away from the tangle as possible. Section the hair.

When to Wet the Hair with Oil

If the core tangle in your hair now looks as though it can be removed with a comb, or if you have removed the majority of the tangles, or if the tangle consists of old hair and dust, this is what you can do: moisten or wet the hair with oils or oil-based products that you might use for conditioning, such as olive oil, coconut oil, castor oil, wheat germ oil, almond oil, avocado oil or any natural oil of your choice.

Because oil can be greasy, I like to mix it with aloe vera gel. Aloe vera gel counterbalances the greasiness of the oils, and the oils counterbalance the drying effect of the aloe vera gel. In combination, they work well together to moisten and soften the hair.

Before placing anything in your hair, do a patch test to ensure that you do not have any allergic reactions to the products you plan to use.

Use Braids to Continue the Detangling Process

Once the hair has been moistened with water, conditioner and/or oil, continue to detangle it, still using your fingers. Then, unless you have very short hair, you should section your hair, no matter what you have used to moisten it. After the hair has been sectioned, very loosely braid each section. If you can, reduce the size of your sections. For example, if you have already divided your hair into four sections, try to divide each section into two more sections. When you finish, you will have eight sections. Loosely braid each section.

Sometimes I braid my hair from the root to the very tips, and sometimes I leave the ends of the hair free. In both cases, the ends of the hair have to be detangled again before styling. You may want to experiment and determine what is best for you.

How Does the Grow It Way of Detangling
Help to Preserve the Structure of the Hair Shaft?

Detangling, which is Step 1 in the Grow It model, minimizes damage to the hair shaft by avoiding unnecessary stress to your hair. This method of detangling does not use mechanical implements, such as brushes or combs, at this step; it uses only your fingers. With enough pressure and force, combs and brushes can strip and rake away the cuticles of the hair shaft. Even worse, if you have product build-up from gels or styling aids, using a comb or brush on hardened hair is almost sure to cause stress, if not breakage, to your precious hair as you forcibly try to separate the product-coated hairs from one another.

Your fingers may pull the hairs, but they are less likely to strip the cuticle structure than a brush or comb would be. Finger combing and detangling minimize the stress and force that you put on your hair as you groom. Therefore, detangling with your fingers aids in the preservation of the hair shaft structure.

Remember, our sole purpose is to try to preserve the structure of the hair shaft, keeping it undamaged for as long as possible—ideally, for the entire life of each strand of hair. By having you detangle first with your fingers, the Grow It model minimizes the damage done during detangling and thus increases your chances of preserving the structure of your hair strands. I am not saying that using a comb or brush to detangle will guarantee damage to the hair shaft; I am saying that the use of the comb and brush at this step increases the likelihood that the hair shaft will be damaged. Since you want to preserve the structure of the hair shaft as long as possible, why should you take a chance of increasing the wear and tear on your hair?

Remember, it is what you do or don't do to your hair that affects its health. Minimizing the use of a comb or brush during the detangling step counts as something you do to preserve the structure of your hair shaft.

Now you can move to Step 2 of the process: Cleansing.

CHAPTER 10

Step 2

All About Cleansing

The term pH is used to measure the acidity or alkalinity of a solution. The pH scale measures the concentration of hydrogen ions in a solution. The "p" stands for potential and the "H" stands for hydrogen. On the pH scale of zero to fourteen, seven is neutral. Hair and skin have a pH of five; lemon juice has a pH of around two; and vinegar of around three. Ideally, when cleansing your hair, you want to use a shampoo or cleanser with a pH that is close to the pH of hair.

The point is that you should use a cleansing agent that does not create too acidic or too alkaline an environment for the hair. High pH shampoos and cleansers may dry out the hair and make it porous. "Porous" simply means that the cuticle is lifted and is no longer lying tight and flat against the hair strand. The result is that the hair strand cannot retain moisture as well as it should; it also cannot keep moisture out as well as it should. If you do use a high pH shampoo, then you will want to use a lower pH, or more acid, conditioner to counterbalance the effects of the shampoo.

As with everything, the key is to find and maintain a balance. That is why the more you understand, the better able you will be able to diagnose the needs of your own hair and to seek out the products, treatments and processes that you require to get your hair healthy and keep it healthy.

Commercial shampoos tend to be water-based. This means that their main ingredient is water. Their second most abundant ingredient is a surfactant (detergent). Surfactant molecules have a hydrophilic front end, which means that the front part of the molecule is attracted to water (hydro), and a lipophilic back end, which means that the back part is attracted to oil (lipo). The attractive force in the surfactant molecule causes oil, dirt and other particles on the hair to ball or bead together. These little balls or beads are then lifted and rinsed away by water, along with the residual shampoo.

I try not to use shampoos that contain surfactants. Some examples of surfactants are lauramide DEA, synthetic lauryl alcohol and laureth 1-40. This is not an exhaustive list. Take a trip to the store and browse through the products, studying their labels. You may also want to purchase a dictionary of cosmetics or hair care product ingredients Use the dictionary to help you determine what surfactants if any, are in the product. Most cosmetic dictionaries will list the names of several surfactants commonly found in shampoos. There are many variations. Therefore I have not provided an exhaustive list. Since it is your hair I encourage you to do the surfactant detection work for yourself.

Weekly Hair Cleansing

If you are using a shampoo to cleanse your hair, pour one to two caps or as much as you need into a cup, glass or bowl. Add warm water to the shampoo and mix thoroughly. Make enough to ensure that your hair will get clean. (I do not recommend storing shampoo once you have diluted it. Most commercial shampoos are made with de-ionized water, or purified water, which has had the minerals and other impurities removed. Nothing in this treated water can interfere with the ions or other components of the shampoo. However, if you add water from your home, which is not likely to be de-ionized, or purified, it could destabilize the product over time.)

Saturate your hair with the soapy water. Squeeze the soapy water through the braids. The physical action from your hands will ensure that the molecules of the surfactant or cleansing agent reaches all the strands of hair within the braids. Repeat as necessary until you believe that your hair is clean.

You might think that it is not possible to get hair clean while it is loosely braided. However, you can clean your loosely braided hair very thoroughly. Therefore, after your hair has been detangled, sectioned and loosely braided, keep it braided for the cleansing part of the process. Only very short hair should be left loose.

When your hair is clean, rinse the cleansing product from the loosely braided sections with water. Don't worry if the braids come a little loose, but don't let them loosen completely.

Using Soap-Based Shampoos to Cleanse the Hair

Soap-based shampoos (unlike shampoos that contain surfactants, or detergents) are made from organic ingredients, such as coconut oil, olive oil or palm oil. Unlike surfactant-based shampoos, soap-based shampoos are dependent on the hardness or softness of the water to create lather and work successfully.

Soft water contains fewer minerals than hard water. The greater quantity of minerals in hard water limits the lathering ability of soap-based shampoos. This is why soap-based shampoos used with hard water may leave more build-up on your hair than surfactant-based shampoos. Lemon juice or vinegar, both of which are considered organic acid rinses, can remove the build-up naturally. Use these rinses after you shampoo with soap.

Using Powders to Cleanse the Hair

If you are using powders to clean your hair, such as those in the Ayuverdic tradition, or even powders from your kitchen, such as baking soda, please first mix these with water in a separate container, just as with shampoo. Once these powders have been mixed with water and placed in the hair, they are not to be manipulated. This means that you should not rub, move or scrub your hair once you place a powder in the hair, as this may cause breakage and/or damage. Please follow the directions provided by the manufacturer of the products you select.

You can also mix your powders with a conditioner instead of water. Think of the powder as an additive to your base conditioner, and follow the instructions below.

Details on Ayurvedic products are outside the scope of this book. Please consult an Ayurvedic beauty book or site for details on these products.

Using a Conditioner to Cleanse the Hair

It is possible to use conditioner instead of shampoo for cleansing. This is called a conditioner wash. Some conditioners contain surfactants, or detergents, so watch out for them if your goal is to eliminate surfactants from your regimen.

To perform a conditioner wash, wet the hair, put conditioner directly in your hair, and use it just like shampoo. There is no need to mix the conditioner with water first, though. Use it straight from the bottle. Be aware that Afro-textured hair may require more than the dime-sized amount suggested by the manufacturer, so feel free to use as much conditioner as you need. Remember, with conditioner washes, the conditioner is used in place of shampoo.

You can mix your conditioner with an oil of your choice if you want your hair to have more lubrication. Pour the conditioner into a cup or container and add a little bit of oil. For a half-cup of conditioner, add approximately one tablespoon of oil. How much oil you use depends upon your choice. Work this mixture through your hair by squeezing your braids in your hands. You may also add cleansing Ayurvedic powders to your conditioner.

Monthly Hair Cleansing

Monthly hair cleansing, or deep cleansing, is important for Afro-textured hair. Monthly hair cleansing is the type of cleansing you need if you want to strip the product build-up from your hair. No matter what types of products you use, whether they are commercial or homemade, synthetic or natural, over time and with continued regular use they all leave build-up on the hair. Therefore, you need to make a special effort to remove the build-up on a regular basis. It is up to you to determine the best time to perform this process on your hair.

For General Clarifying

Once a month, use a shampoo or product that is specifically meant for clarifying the hair. These clarifying products will leave the hair squeaky clean. They literally strip your hair of the build-up of other products, but they can strip it of its natural oils, too. Not everybody can use every clarifying shampoo; some people cannot use clarifying shampoo, or even regular shampoo, at all. Each individual must determine what works best for her.

To Prepare for Specific Treatments

Another reason to perform a monthly cleansing that is different from your weekly cleansing is to prepare the hair to better receive special treatments, such as deep protein treatments, deep moisturizing treatments, deep conditioning treatments and straightening processes.

Straightening processes here include hot comb presses, flat iron presses and blow-drying. They do not include any kind of chemical process, such as a partial or full permanent relaxing. Hair that is to be permanently relaxed should be bathed in moisture, but not in oil or grease, every day for at least a week or two prior to the relaxing treatment to nurture and to fortify it.

Hair will absorb treatments better after it has been rinsed with a diluted solution of apple cider vinegar and water. If you decide to use vinegar, mix a capful or two with several cups of water. However, remember that apple cider vinegar is highly acidic, and it can be hard on dry, fragile hair and relaxed hair. Use it only infrequently, no more than once a month. Determining the proportion of apple cider vinegar and the level of acidity your hair can take may be another trial-and-error process that you may have to follow.

How Does the Grow It Way of Cleansing Help to Preserve the Structure of the Hair Shaft?

Dirt and oil on unclean hair can cause the hair to stick together and weigh it down. The Grow It model minimizes the wear and tear on your hair. It allows you to disperse the cleansing product evenly throughout your hair, and less manipulation and effort will be needed to spread and remove the cleanser. It ensures that the bulk of your hair is flowing in the natural direction: downward and away from your scalp. It minimizes tangling.

The Grow It model of cleansing provides three distinct benefits:

1. It keeps the hair from becoming more tangled during cleansing. This offsets or helps to decrease the need to detangle at every step in the Grow It Process.

2. It allows you to ensure that your hair strands are smoothed in the same direction. Smoothing constantly and gently ensures that the cuticles of the hair are encouraged to flow in their natural direction: away from the scalp and downward to your neck or back.

3. It allows you to aim your diluted shampoo or hair cleanser at the scalp, where cleansing action is most needed. Applying the less concentrated product to a single area of your head means that you will not be spending lots of time trying to move your hair around to get the product to other areas, or to get it completely out of the hair.

In the Grow It model of cleansing, you can vigorously squeeze the cleanser through your braided or plaited hair without creating significant tangling. When cleansing loose hair, the individual strands are likely to flow in different directions and become tangled. Sectioning the hair in loose braids and cleansing it with diluted cleanser aids in the preservation of the hair shaft structure because it keeps the bulk of the hair flowing in the natural direction of the cuticle structure, which is downward.

The fewer tangles you have, the less detangling you need to perform. The less detangling you need to perform, the less stress you place upon your hair strands. The less stress you place upon your hair strands, the less likely you are to strip cuticles or break hair. Clean, unbroken hair, smoothed in the direction of the natural flow of the hair cuticle structure, is comparable to the untouched state of your natural hair. Cleansing this way counts as something you should do, as it preserves the structure of your hair shaft.

Now you can move to Step 3, which is all about conditioning.

CHAPTER 11

Step 3

All About Conditioning

*H*air is said to be triboelectric, which means that when it is rubbed it generates an electrical charge. The electrical charge generated by hair is negative. This negative electrical charge can be created when hair rubs against other hair, clothing, furniture, or even against one's own skin.

The molecules of most conditioning agents carry small positive electrical charges. The negative charge in the hair attracts these positively charged molecules. The positive molecules are then deposited on the hair, especially where there are damaged, chipped, or missing cuticle layers. The positive and negative charges cancel each other out, reducing static electricity in the hair.

Static electricity can leave hair with a dry, fly-away look. Conditioners alleviate this.

The best way to avoid split ends is to use conditioning as a proactive, preventive measure to keep damage at bay. Conditioners also help the raised cuticle scales to lie flat against the hair shaft. This smoothes the strand and prevents it from catching on other hair. One function of healthy, tightly flattened, intact cuticles is that they reflect light. Therefore, conditioned hair has improved luster and shine.

It is important to avoid all thermal straightening treatments, such as pressing, blow-drying and flat ironing. If you want to do the maximum toward preserving your natural hair structure, you should also avoid all chemical treatments, such as permanent waving, relaxing, texlaxing and dyeing.

Wetting the hair opens up the cuticle scales on the hair. It can also make the hair swell. When the cuticle scales are lifted and left open, the surface of the hair feels rough. Lifted cuticles become weathered or damaged more quickly than cuticles that have not been lifted. Therefore, it is important to use conditioner in your hair on a regular basis. Remember, even if you are keeping your hair totally natural, the hair is wet at all times. Wet hair can have lifted, or swollen, cuticles.

Some type of conditioning agent is necessary to preserve the natural structure of your hair. Look for protein extracts such as panthenol, collagen, silk protein and amino acids in your conditioning products.

A Word on Loosely Woven Braids

People believe that if their hair is cleansed or conditioned in braids, they cannot get the full benefits of the treatment. However, if done correctly, I think it is possible to benefit from performing these treatments with the hair loosely braided. You can thoroughly clean and condition your hair while it is in loose braids.

Once you understand that the purpose of your routine is to preserve the structure of your hair strands, it is not difficult to see the benefits of keeping the hair braided for cleansing and conditioning. By keeping the hair braided, you are employing several beneficial actions. First, you detangle your hair without using a comb or brush. These styling tools can strip the precious cuticle structure. Second, you smooth the hair before braiding it. This ensures that the cuticles are all flowing in their natural, downward direction, away from the scalp. Third, the braids allow you to minimize the manipulation of your hair during washing or conditioning, keeping the creation of new tangles to a minimum. Finally, wet hair can be damaged by friction. The action of gently squeezing the braids as you clean and condition reduces this friction. For the same reason, I do not recommend that you vigorously towel-dry your hair. Towel drying creates too much friction and opportunity to seriously damage your hair.

Many people recommend that you should wash and condition your hair in the bathtub. I do not recommend that you perform your hair processes while you are sitting in the bathtub, because the soft tissues on our bodies can become irritated if we sit in the water and expose them to hair products, whether they are natural or synthetic. Many people suggest that you wash your hair in the shower, because they feel that you can get your hair cleaner more quickly and free of product more easily under the steady stream of the shower. Also, in the shower you can also keep your hair flowing in the same direction. I personally prefer to wash my hair in the sink, which accomplishes the same goals.

No matter where you choose to wash and condition your hair, the key thing is that you should always section your hair into four to eight braids, whether your hair is short or long. If the braids are kept loose near the scalp and all down the braid, you can rinse your hair by squeezing the braids while running them under water. It might take a little more time than rinsing loose hair, but you are minimizing the manipulation of the individual strands of hair. You can move your braids around your head to add product, cleanse the scalp and rinse. Once you finish cleansing, your hair will not be tangled, as it would if you left it loose.

If you cleanse your hair without braiding it, you have to be careful to minimize the amount of manipulation you do, or you will risk tangling your hair. Thus, you may have to rub your scalp less vigorously with the pads of your fingers than you can if your hair is braided. This is why I recommend cleansing hair that is loosely braided rather than completely loosened.

Even if your hair is short, get into the habit of braiding it. The Grow It Process is about gaining health, and ultimately retaining more length in your natural hair. If you are already in the habit of braiding your hair for the cleansing and conditioning process, that is one less thing you have to learn, think about and remember to do. When your hair starts to gain length—and it will—you will not be overwhelmed when you decide to wash and condition your longer, natural Afro-textured hair.

The test of a good, solid hair care regimen is that it is put together conscientiously with lots of thought and care. It should be simple enough to be performed regularly on autopilot once it is firmly entrenched in your brain.

A Word on the Importance of Smoothing

It is important to smooth Afro-textured hair in the same direction constantly as you begin to condition. The direction should be away and downward from your scalp. This can be done simply by taking a section of hair, whether braided or loose, gently grasping it in your hand and pulling your hand down over the braid or section of hair several times to smooth it out.

Smoothing should be done for two reasons. The first reason is connected with conditioning. You condition your hair to help smooth the cuticles, with the result that the hair feels smoother and softer to the touch after the conditioning treatment. Even though smoothing with your hands does not flatten the hair cuticle, it helps the conditioning process by arranging all the hair in one direction. Also, your hands become familiar with how your hair feels, and if something is amiss—if you are using a product that is not good for your hair, or if there is a change in your hair—you will be able to recognize it quickly because your hands remember how your hair should feel. Smoothing adds information and data to your hair model. By smoothing before, during and after conditioning, you can better gauge whether or not the conditioner you have selected is beneficial for your hair. If the hair is still in a roughened state after you have conditioned it, the conditioner that you have chosen is not helping to preserve the structure of the hair; it is not helping to lay the cuticles flat against the hair strand. Or the shampoo that you used may have been too alkaline or too drying for your hair type; it may have lifted the cuticles. Smoothing is a way to gather clues to help you better analyze the state and the needs of your hair.

Hair Jump

The second reason for smoothing is something that I call hair jump. Hair jump is the amazing athleticism of Afro-textured hair. It can spring up high, from waist to neck, in a single bound. Many people refer to this as hair shrinkage, but I don't think that phrase captures the amazing versatility and character of Afro-textured hair. This is what hair jump refers to.

In its natural state, Afro-textured hair can draw itself up and hang to only one-third of its actual length, or even shorter. Sometimes it can curl so much that it hangs five times shorter than the length it has when it is straightened or manually pulled straight. While it is true that other ethnic groups also have curly hair, Afro-textured hair in particular can curl up naturally into tight coils and jump great distances with a single pull or tug. That is why some types of Afro-textured hair can hold the most beautiful braided and twisted styles for long periods of time without having to be taken down and redone.

If your hair is natural, it can have an incredible jump. For example, your natural hair may draw up to your neck, but if you pull it with your fingers or have it straightened with heat, that same hair might reach from your neck all the way down to your waist. Because of this super coiling ability, Afro-textured hair can become easily tangled. One wrong move and you could lose a beautiful, precious lock of coiled hair forever.

Conditioning your hair the right way is one of the most critical steps in the Grow It Process. This is because it is at this point, after having conditioned your hair, that I suggest that you pick up your comb to fully and thoroughly detangle your hair. If there is one step where you should take your time, this is it. Your hair is now completely wet, which means that it is in its most vulnerable natural state, and you are about to put tension on your hair to detangle it. You should take great care and time with this step.

Conditioner Comb-Out

If your hair has a lot of product build-up, leaving conditioner in can make the hair gummy or sticky. If your hair feels gummy or sticky, you may want to give your braided hair an extra rinse under warm running water. Squeeze each braid with your fingers and hands. You should be able to feel whether the hair is still gummy.

There is no need to completely rinse all the conditioner out of your hair completely. Try to keep enough conditioner in to create an environment in which your wide-tooth comb can move through your hair without getting stuck and immobilized because of too much product.

Move the other braids away from the braid on which you are going to be working. You can use a nylon knee-high as a ponytail holder to anchor all the braids except the one you are working on. Once you have isolated one braid from the others, unbraid it.

Now smooth the loosened hair with your hands and fingers, so that you do not create unnecessary tangles. Once you have smoothed the hair, the three sections that made up the braid are all together in one section. Grasp the hair in the middle of the section, place the comb below your hand and about two inches above the very ends of the hair, and gently comb it through to the ends. When the comb runs smoothly through those two inches, grasp the section again, this time about an inch higher up, leaving a longer stretch of hair hanging free, and again comb through to the ends. Keep performing this process until you have combed through the entire section, from the scalp to the hair ends.

Once you have detangled this section, you can loosely braid it up again to keep it tangle-free. Move on to the next braid and repeat the same actions. When you have gone through your entire head, unbraiding, combing and re-braiding, you can rinse all your loosely braided hair under running water. Have your towel handy so that you can wrap it over your head and squeeze the braids to remove the excess water.

How Does the Grow It Way of Conditioning
Help to Preserve the Structure of the Hair Shaft?

Conditioning helps smooth the cuticles of the hair shaft in one direction. It gets you in the habit of regularly examining your hair, so that you can anticipate its needs before you start to see any damage.

In the Grow It Process, you are asked to make conscious decisions about the state and needs of your hair. The Grow It model prompts you to think about the conditioner you select each time, basing your choice upon the needs of your hair on the day you are using the conditioner. Does your hair need moisture? If so, it would benefit from a moisturizing conditioner. Does it require protein? Then it would benefit from a protein conditioner.

The main importance of the Grow It method of conditioning is that it gets you into the habit of proactively and consciously examining your hair. This examination trains you to learn about the state of your hair so that you understand how to address its needs at the time of the examination, apart from and independent of anyone else. This knowledge will empower you to make good decisions even while you still entrust your hair to your favorite hair care professional. Your hair is ever-changing. You want to get into the habit of performing this examination in anticipation of your hair needs, not after you start to see damage.

The act of conditioning the sectioned, loosely braided hair further increases your ability to smooth your hair in the natural direction and flow of the cuticle structure. Cuticles that are lying flat prevent excess moisture from leeching away from the inner structure of the hair, prevent excess water from entering the inner core of the hair, and help it better reflect light. Thus, properly conditioned hair, in which the cuticle structure is encouraged to lie flat, has a better shine. In addition, conditioner serves as a lubricant, decreasing the friction between individual hairs. The less friction on the hair, the less likely it is that one strand or a few will cut or saw across other strands and damage them.

Many people with Afro-textured hair can add natural oils to the conditioning product, to increase the lubricating effect of the conditioner. Adding oil to your conditioner is optional, not required. Some hair and products do well with the addition of oil, others do not. You need to make that determination for yourself.

Depending upon how the conditioner is formulated, conditioning can decrease the flyaway look in your hair. Some conditioners are formulated to add moisture, and some are formulated to strengthen hair, usually by adding protein. This helps you to have hair that is less frizzy and dry after you wash, condition and groom it. Conditioning your hair every time you wash it counts as something you should do in order to preserve the structure of your hair shaft.

Now you are ready to move to Step 4, which is all about moisturizing.

CHAPTER 12

Step 4

All About Moisturizing

The entire routine and process of your personal hair care should be aimed at preventing injury to your hair. By caring for your hair and nurturing it, you will be better able to preserve the structure of your hair. Everything you do should be done with thought and care, and as gently as possible.

Step 4 of the Grow It Process is keeping the hair moisturized. To see why it is important to keep hair moisturized, it is important to understand the tendency of Afro-textured hair to be dry and to know what types of actions exacerbate this condition, or what makes dry hair even drier.

The Tendency toward Dryness

Hair that is perpetually dry will eventually end up damaged. Hair that is damaged will split. Hair that is split will end up breaking. Breaking hair does not retain growth. Growth that is not retained results in hair that either never seems to grow past a certain length, or keeps breaking and getting shorter, or is always dull and unhealthy looking. Continuous dryness is the biggest enemy of any hair. It is especially detrimental for natural Afro-textured hair.

What exactly is dry hair? Dry hair is hair that does not contain enough moisture. This definition is independent of the argument about whether the dryness is due to heredity or environment. The point is that whatever the cause, it is possible to address dry hair and improve its appearance. If your hair is currently damaged beyond recovery, but you still have new hair emerging and growing from your scalp—meaning that you are not bald—you can address and improve the issue of dry hair with knowledge, proper care and handling and use of the right products.

Weathering

Weathering is the gradual wearing away of the cuticle. Because of this damage, the cortex becomes exposed. The cortex, as well as the cuticle, is then worn away. Eventually the hair splits, and ultimately it breaks.

Weathering is a natural process that has little effect on the hair all at once. It is cumulative: it occurs because of actions or experiences that are repeated over time. It is speeded up, or expedited, by what you do to your hair.

The following all cause weathering: wetting hair; friction on the hair; sunlight; heat from dryers and styling implements; chemicals in the bath, shower or pool water; salt and minerals in sea water; as well as cosmetic procedures. These all contribute to the rapid weathering of the hair. Weathering is also affected by what you do not do. Not using conditioner on a regular basis, for example, is not taking an action; this will result in your hair becoming weathered faster.

The ends of the hair may look lighter in color than the rest because of normal weathering. This affects everyone's hair. Heavily weathered hair tends to look even lighter; it has a white or grayish cast on the ends. Hair that is severely weathered also tends to be brittle.

Bonds of the Hair

The hair is made of several types of bonds, located in the cortex of the hair strand. The bonds are hydrogen, salt, disulfide and peptide bonds. Hydrogen, salt and disulfide bonds each account for one-third of the overall strength of the hair. Hydrogen and salt bonds are far more numerous than disulfide bonds; disulfide bonds are the strongest of the three.

Hydrogen bonds. These are physical bonds. The hydrogen bond is a side bond, located on the side of the polypeptide chain. It helps hold one side of the polypeptide chain to the side of another polypeptide chain. Polypeptide chains are amino acid chains linked by disulfide bonds. Disulfide bonds are very strong and are discussed in detail later in this chapter. Hydrogen bonds account for some of the overall strength of the hair.

Physical bonds that have been changed can be returned to their original state. The hydrogen bond is a weak, temporary physical bond, which can be broken by water or heat. The hydrogen bond is affected when you apply heat to your hair to straighten it, or when you wet your hair and sit under a dryer in order to obtain a curly wet set. The bond can be reformed, or returned to its original state, by drying or cooling the hair.

Salt bonds. These, too, are physical bonds. Like the hydrogen bond, the salt bond is a side bond, located on the side of the polypeptide chain. It helps hold one side of the polypeptide chain to the side of another polypeptide chain, and it accounts for the some of the overall strength of the hair.

The salt bond is a weak physical bond, which can be broken by changes in the pH of the hair. Solutions that are strongly alkaline or strongly acidic will break the salt bond; it can be reformed by normalizing the pH. Using water mixed with lemon juice or vinegar on the hair can strengthen the salt bonds, tightening the cuticle of the hair. Again, the caveat here is that this is the general result. We have discussed earlier what can happen if an acidic solution is just too acidic for your type of hair.

Disulfide bonds. These are chemical bonds. Chemical bonds are stronger than physical bonds, and once they are changed, they cannot be returned to their original state. The strong disulfide bond can be broken by the chemicals used in permanents, permanent relaxers, hydroxide and straightening relaxers. The disulfide bond can be reformed or converted to another type of bond, called a lanthionine bond, but it can never return to its original state. This is the reason why it is not possible to wash or sweat out the relaxer in your hair.

Once the disulfide bonds have been changed, they are permanently changed. Changing these bonds weakens the hair and tends to make it drier than it would be if you had not received the chemical treatment that affects the disulfide bonds.

Healthy looking relaxed hair is not an oxymoron (an oxymoron means a contradiction in terms). It is possible to have relaxed hair that appears healthy, but the care of relaxed hair is beyond the scope of this book. One of the best books on addressing the specific needs of relaxed hair is *Ultra Black Hair Growth II* by Cathy Howse.

Peptide bonds. These are strong chemical bonds. They can be broken by hair removers. Hair removers are also called chemical depilatories. Like the disulfide bonds, once the peptide bonds are broken, they can never be reformed. If a peptide bond is broken, the hair is dissolved. Therefore, remember that when you use hair removal cream, you are breaking the peptide bonds of the hair.

Now that you understand weathering and the different bonds of the hair, it should be clear to you why conditioning the hair is so important and why it is best to avoid chemical treatments if you want to retain as much healthy length as possible. Conditioning can strengthen the hair and help to slow down the effects of weathering. Chemical treatments weaken the hair by breaking down or completely dissolving the bonds of the hair.

The point of this information is to help you make conscious choices that are best for you, your situation and your hair. Natural Afro-textured hair is not for everyone. For some women, the best choice may be a chemical relaxer. Make your hair choices with your eyes wide open. If you do so, you are less likely to regret and agonize over a less-than-thoughtful choice later on.

Damaged hair is weakened hair. As you know, in damaged hair the cuticle begins to break down. Eventually, the cuticle disappears, layer by layer. Then the cortex is exposed, split ends appear and the hair breaks.

Hair tends toward dryness because of the way it is handled. The amount of manipulation of the hair, the external environment, oxidizing chemicals and product overload can all contribute to hair damage.

Damage from Manipulation

Damage from manipulation can be due to poorly sharpened or cheap cutting implements, mechanical implements and heating implements. By themselves, the processes that employ these implements are not bad for your hair, but they must be used in moderation and with thought, with the goal of preserving the sacred structure of the hair while styling.

Scissors and Razors

It is important to use sharp, good-quality stainless steel scissors. These scissors should be made for the sole purpose of cutting hair, and used only for cutting your hair. Any pair of scissors will not do. Sharp, steel scissors cut cleanly. Blunt or dull-edged scissors leave a cut with a long, jagged edge. The jagged edge is the edge of the now damaged cuticle, which will not lie down smoothly. This will allow the cuticle scales to be even further weakened and vulnerable to damage.

Razor cutting, whether the razor is dull or sharpened, produces long, tapering sections of cuticle that weather very quickly. The edges of hair cut with a razor or with cheap or dull scissors can leave the hair ends in such an exposed state that the cuticle may even peel back.

Mechanical Damage

Overuse or vigorous, rough use of brushes and combs are the biggest culprits in causing mechanical damage.

For many women with natural Afro-textured hair, puffs and Afros are favorite styles. If you are making Afro-puffs and Afros by teasing or back-combing your hair, you are lifting the scales of the cuticle and forcing them back in the wrong direction. Just because a style is applied to natural hair does not necessarily mean that the style is good for your hair. If you continue to create these styles by back-combing and teasing without smoothing the hair, you will remove the cuticle scales. This will weaken your hair and make it vulnerable to damage in the form of splits and breakage. You will have compromised your hair and your ability to preserve its structure and extend its life. To gain length, hair has to be around for years. The improper use of brushes and combs can destroy the longevity and health of your hair very quickly.

Heat Damage

Heat damage comes in many forms. It can be caused by the overuse of curling irons, blow dryers, flat irons and/or pressing combs. Using a pressing comb is also referred to as thermal relaxing.

Processes such as blow-drying reduce the moisture content of your hair to below its normal level. In addition, the blow dryer itself can be harmful. Heated appliances soften the keratin, or protein, of the hair. If they are too hot, they can actually cause the water in the hair to boil, making steam bubbles form inside the softened hair shaft. Severely heat-damaged hair must be cut.

Damage from the Environment

Damage from the environment comes from two main sources, sun exposure and wind exposure.

Sun Exposure

Ultraviolet rays from the sun affect the hair similarly to the way hair bleach affects hair. Like bleach, the oxidizing rays from the sun can break down, or change the chemical composition and the components of the hair. Oxidation from the sun causes free radicals to form. Oxygen causes free radicals to break away.

In general, from a chemistry standpoint, the oxidation process is the interaction of oxygen molecules with substances in which they come in contact. In the oxidation process, there is a loss of at least one electron when two substances interact. An electron is a component of an atom. Two or more atoms form a molecule. Molecules form groups. Groups form bonds.

Specifically, hair contains a chemical group called a thiol group. These thiol groups stabilize the hair by forming disulfide bonds. Remember, disulfide bonds are very strong bonds and contribute greatly to the strength of the hair. Thiol groups on the hair make the hair strand slippery and help hairs slide across one another. If the hair is oxidized by the sun, the disulfide bonds then turn into compounds called sulfonic acids. In comparison to thiol groups, sulfonic acids on the hair are sticky. Hair with sulfonic acids, which come from oxidized disulfide bonds, tangles more readily than hair that does not have sulfonic acids on it. The change from disulfide bonds to sulfonic acids is permanent. Lubrication, such as conditioner, can provide more slip for the hair that has sulfonic acids on it, to make it more manageable and to minimize the tangles.

To prevent oxidation caused by oxygen, it is necessary to provide a layer of protection between the exposed material, in our case, the hair strand, and the sun. Creation of free radicals is minimized if exposure of the hair to the sun is minimized. The effects of oxidation can be better managed if the oxygen cannot penetrate the surface of the hair to reach the free radicals. This is why it is important to cover the hair when you are in the sun and to add conditioners to your hair when you are going to be outside in the sun for extended periods of time. Wind exposure can also oxidize the hair.

Wind Exposure (Air)

Exposure to wind or air, too, has an impact on the hair. When the air is very arid (dry), it leeches moisture from the hair. The air also carries pollutants; it serves as a medium that deposits dirt and grime in your hair. Letting the wind whip your hair may look sexy, but is not good for your hair. Blowing strands can rub against each other, creating friction and electrical charges. Wind or air exposure expedites the weathering process and can be slowed down by using protective styling. If you plan to be traveling in an open car or boat, or yacht, tie your hair back and cover it.

Damage from Oxidizing Chemicals

Hair is made up primarily of proteins. Harsh oxidizers chip away at the outer layers of the cuticle and expose the inner layers of the cortex. Several oxidizing chemicals affect hair: chlorine, neutralizers in permanent waving processing and relaxer chemicals. Permanent waving and relaxing are outside the scope of this book and are not addressed here.

Chlorine is a harsh oxidizer. You do not have to be a swimmer to have chlorine-damaged hair. It is found in tap water and in bath and shower water in most homes in the United States. Chlorine can damage the cuticle and proteins of the hair. It can worsen the oxidizing effects of the air and sun, and thus worsen the conditions of the hair. Chlorine can cause hair to become brittle and to lack shine. Chlorine has a positive charge and is attracted to negatively charged hair.

Damage from Minerals

Water with lots of minerals is defined as hard water. Hard water can cause mineral build-up on your hair: the resins from styling products, such as shampoos, conditioners, gels and leave-in products, attach to the minerals in the water. This creates dull, dry hair. Generally, a person reacts to this by piling on more products to combat the dullness, thus falling even deeper down the rabbit hole of dull, dry, damaged hair. Minerals have a positive charge and are attracted to negatively charged hair.

Whether you are using hard water in your home or you are bathing or swimming in the sea, there are minerals in the water that affect your hair. The salt in seawater can be very drying. Combined with the ocean breeze and the rays of the sun, this will expedite the oxidation of your hair. Tap water that is unfiltered or has not gone through a softening process may contain magnesium and other minerals. As mentioned already, water that contains these minerals is called hard water. The minerals in hard water affect the ability of soap-based cleansers to form lather, and they can damage the hair directly. Magnesium can dry the hair; it can coat the hair, causing it to appear weighted down and flat; it can inhibit the proper processing of permanent waving, coloring and relaxing; and it can cause the hair to lack shine.

The minerals in the water can combine with the products you use and build up on the hair, leaving it coated and dull. One way to offset the effect of minerals in the water is to install a water filter in your bath or shower. There are many kinds of filters that can be purchased, ranging from inexpensive to costly ones.

Damage from Product Overload

Product build-up can make the hair appear dull and dry. If the ingredients of a hair care product do not agree with your hair type, they can leech moisture from the hair and move it toward dryness. Product resins can become sticky and harden on the hair. These resins attract more product, and the build-up can cause breakage if you then try to comb or brush your hair.

Now that we have examined how hair can be made drier, and how dry hair can lead to damaged hair, let's proceed to Step 4 of the Grow It Process: moisturizing the hair.

Moisturizing the Hair

Even though hair can absorb moisture from the environment, it is not always possible to determine and control the state of your environment. We know that in general, Afro-textured hair tends toward dryness. You can anticipate this by actively moisturizing your hair to combat dryness and keep damage to a minimum. The way to do this is to add moisture to your hair on a regular basis.

Moisturize According to Whether Your Hair Is Curly or Straightened

If your hair is curly, meaning it is in its natural state, a water-based moisturizer may be a good option for you. If your hair is straightened, a lotion-type of moisturizer, or one with very little water, may work best.

Natural (Curly) Hair

When your hair is in its natural state, water-based products can help to keep it moisturized. Examples of these water-based products are curl activators and inexpensive, conditioner-based concoctions that you mix yourself. You can mix simple, basic concoctions or more complex ones.

Basic Concoction

To make a basic moisturizing concoction, purchase an inexpensive spray bottle from a beauty supply store or a grocery store. Fill the bottle halfway with inexpensive, water-based hair conditioner. Then thin it out by adding some water to the bottle. Lastly, you can add one-quarter cup to one-half cup of oil, such as olive, sesame or castor, to your mixture. This spray is relatively easy to make, and it can be used daily.

Complex Concoction

To the basic moisturizing concoction mentioned above, you can add 3-5 drops each of two or three essential oils, such as oil of rosemary, cedar wood, lavender, peppermint, sage or basil. Remember, in the case of essential oils, more is not necessarily better. Be sure that you are selecting unadulterated essential oils and not fragrance oils. Essential oils are natural oils; fragrance oils are manufactured and loaded with synthetic perfumes.

Panthenol, the Moisture Master

Panthenol, derived from vitamin B, provides moisture. It is absorbed into the hair shaft, and it penetrates the scalp and reaches the hair follicle underneath the scalp. Panthenol improves the moisture content of the hair as soon as the hair starts to grow. Look for panthenol in your product ingredients.

Consider incorporating a panthenol-heavy product in the moisturizing component of your hair routine, such as in your daily moisturizer. You can buy panthenol from websites that carry cosmetic ingredients, but it is easier to start with a panthenol-heavy product. Even though panthenol is considered a great moisturizer, it does not work well for everyone, and you will incur less risk and investment if you buy a panthenol-based product off the store shelf, rather than ordering it online and paying extra for shipping.

Straightened Hair

Natural hair that has been straightened will revert to its curly or kinky state if water-based moisture is placed on or in the hair. Therefore, to provide moisture, it is advisable to use a lotion-type moisturizer on straightened hair. These products have water in them, but the amount of water they contain and the way in which they are formulated allow them to be placed on straightened hair without making it revert to its curly state.

Oil-based moisturizes can be placed on the very ends of the hair, near the hairline and the nape of the neck. Different people have different types of hair, as well as different product preferences. One product doesn't work for everyone. Each person has to find what works best for her and her hair.

Sealing In Moisture by Using Head Coverings

One way to seal in the moisture that you put into your hair is to use head coverings. The best types of head coverings are made of plastic, satin, silk and nylon, as these materials will not leech the moisture from your hair. Cotton, although it is natural, it is not the best choice for maintaining the moisture content in Afro-textured hair, because cotton tends to absorb moisture.

Plastic Head Coverings

Plastic is inexpensive and readily available, but is not necessarily good for the environment. Two types of plastic coverings that can be used are plastic shower caps and plastic sandwich bags. Plastic shower caps can be worn under whole-head wigs and at night, when you retire. Please do not wear a shower cap in public unless you cover it with a hat or kerchief. This is in poor taste and not at all attractive.

The two methods of using plastic head coverings are described as the whole-head baggie method and the section or ponytail baggie method.

Whole-Head Baggie Method

This method works for both very short and very long hair. Take a plastic bag or cap and place it over your moisturized hair. The whole-head baggie or plastic cap can be worn for a few hours during the day or evening, or it can be secured over your head for the duration of the night, until the next morning. This is not recommended when your hair is wet and the climate is cold. You don't want to get sick!

Section or Ponytail Baggie Method

This method works best when you have enough hair to pull back into a ponytail. Try to find the inexpensive plastic sandwich bags, ones that do not have a locking seal but require some kind of tie to seal them. The ties should be included with the plastic bags; these types of bags work very well. Place a water-based moisturizer on your hair, or an oil-based moisturizer on the ends of your hair. Braid or twist your hair or wrap it in a bun, and then place the bag over the braided or twisted hair. Or you can simply stuff your loose hair into the bag and secure the bag around your hair with a nylon knee-high. You can leave the bag on overnight or wear it during the day underneath another knee-high, a phony ponytail, or a scarf or hat.

Satin Head Coverings

Satin head coverings can be inexpensive, but more costly than plastic. Satin scarves are far more interesting than plastic, though, because you can purchase them in a variety of colors and styles from the grocery store or beauty supply store. Satin scarves can be employed in several ways. The two methods that I use the most are the whole-head method and the section or ponytail method, outlined below.

There is no separate section for the use of silk or nylon. I sometimes use nylon in conjunction with a satin scarf. You can make a nylon base by cutting the seat of a pair of pantyhose. Place it over your hair and cover it with silk or satin. Now proceed to the satin scarf methods below.

Whole-Head Satin Scarf Method

This method works well to protect the hair from rubbing against cotton sheets and clothing. For day wear, wrap the satin scarf around your head and wear it under a hat. You can also put a wig over the scarf, but the scarf wrapped around your head might be too bulky to accommodate certain wigs and head shapes. For night wear, wrap the scarf securely enough so that it will not fall off your head during sleep. Satin scarves help straightened hair to maintain its shine, and they prevent it from becoming too dry. Satin scarves work better with oil-based moisturizers. Water-based moisturizers tend to saturate the satin, staining the scarves and everything they touch.

Section or Ponytail Satin Scarf Method

Simply wrap the scarf around the ponytail. A scarf will stay on a twisted or braided ponytail better than on a ponytail with the ends flowing loosely.

You might argue that using plastic bags and scarves on your head does not really belong in the section on moisturizing but in the section on protecting, which follows. It really depends upon your perspective. Because these methods of covering the head are closely connected with the application of moisturizer, I have included them here.

How Does the Grow It Way of Moisturizing Help to Preserve the Structure of the Hair Shaft?

Whether or not they contain oil and other additional emollients, water-based leave-in products preserve the hair structure by adding moisture to the hair shaft. This helps to increase the suppleness and flexibility of the hair strand. Supple, moisturized hair is more likely to be pliable and soft, to lie and bend. Hair that is not moisturized is more likely to be hard and brittle and to break under the stress of everyday grooming.

Wetting the hair frequently during the week is also a way to keep hair moist. Previously, in the section on weathering, I mentioned that wetting the hair caused weathering. Wetting and drying the hair causes the breaking and reformation of the bonds and linkages of the hair. This breaking and reforming of bonds and linkages does add to the wear and tear of hair. But, as with all things one must strike a balance. In the case of hair the way balance is struck is to understand that by using water, this keeps hair moist and pliable and alleviates chronic dryness. It is important to understand that chronically dry hair will become damaged and weather faster than wetting and drying your hair naturally. However, wetting and drying your hair with artificial heat from such tools as blow dryers and hair dryers will weather your hair the fastest. Thus, even though wetting the hair can lead to it being weathered, the overall benefit is that it keeps the hair moist. The true culprit and helpmate of weathering is chronic dryness. You really want to avoid having chronically dry hair.

If you choose to wet your hair every day, it is important to use a water filter on your shower and/or in your bath. If you don't, you could be defeating the purpose of frequently wetting the hair. This is because you could be increasing the number of times you are exposing your hair and scalp to chlorine, other chemicals and mineral-laden water, all of which can dry the hair.

Perpetually dry hair tends to wear out faster. Afro-textured hair that is completely natural and never receives any color and/or heat treatments still requires that moisture be applied to it in some form or another.

Let's move on to Step 5, which is all about protecting.

CHAPTER 13

Step 5

All About Protecting

It is always a good idea to protect your hair with scarves, coverings and specific styling methods. The limitation of this type of protection is that you are only addressing the symptom; obviously, the protection only lasts as long as the covering is kept on the hair.

Strengthening Your Hair

The best way to protect your hair is to strengthen it. You can employ various internal and external methods to strengthen your hair.

Strengthen Internally

Good food and clean water are two internal components to which you should pay attention. I am not a big vitamin user, and I don't take them on a regular basis. However, when I do take them, usually in two-week spurts, I tend to see a difference in my skin and hair.

Good Food

Good food, such as raw vegetables and fruits and organic, unprocessed foods are ideal for the health of your body and hair. A balanced diet filled with organic vegetable juices and raw fruits gives your body excellent nutrition. Remove and permanently eliminate as many re-fined and processed foods from your diet as possible.

Water

Try to find the water that's best for you. If you don't like bottled water, don't drink it. If you prefer filtered water, drink that. Try to have water every day. Please do not agonize over which water is best; just up your intake.

Vitamins

There are certain vitamins that are recommended for hair. First, if possible, try to find a whole food multi-vitamin. They can be found at health food stores and online. In addition to the whole food multi-vitamin, biotin and vitamin B complex for stress are recommended for the hair. Please perform your own research prior to instituting and implementing your vitamin regimen.

Managing Stress, Deep Breathing and Exercise

Stress can eat away at your health, your hair and your progress. Stress can work against you by creating internal havoc. In extreme cases, stress can create chemical imbalances and hair loss. Also, when under stress you are more likely not to take the time to work on your hair.

When you are under stress, it is important to manage the stress as best you can. Maintain your nutrient balance through good food, and supplement it with vitamins. But remember, vitamins cannot replace good food. Deep breathing and exercise help to keep the body in bal-ance. This indirectly affects the health of your hair.

Strengthen Externally

Using protein treatments, deep conditioning treatments and leave-ins are external ways to strengthen and protect your hair.

Protein Treatments

Two kinds of protein treatments can protect your hair: light protein and heavy protein. These distinctions are arbitrary. There is no product called a light protein or heavy protein treatment. The terms have been applied here to distinguish between the two types of products, to help you better determine what may work best for you at any given time.

Light Protein Treatments

I consider light protein treatments to be protein treatments that require you to place them on your hair for only a few minutes and then rinse them out. These types of products tend to use words like "re-constructor" or "protein treatment" on the label. Light protein treatments can be used on a frequent basis, such as weekly.

Curl activators, which are often made with wheat, soy or hydrolyzed animal proteins, are another form of light protein treatment. Curl activators are leave-ins, as they are not rinsed out of your hair once they are applied. They can be used daily.

Heavy Protein Treatments

Heavy protein treatments require that you place them in your hair and add heat from a source such as a hair dryer or blow dryer. Some of these heavy protein treatments are designed to harden on the hair. They should be rinsed out.

The key to these heavier protein treatments is that they must be used with heat to be effective. These treatments should not be used too frequently, only once every six to eight weeks.

Some of the heavy protein treatments are to be used on damaged hair. However, in my case, these heavier protein treatments, used proactively, have served to protect my hair, enabling me to reach longer lengths with fewer split ends. You do not have to have damaged hair to use these heavy protein treatments.

Protein products are said to rebuild the structure of the hair by replacing essential proteins that have been stripped away by daily styling implements and products. They use activated proteins combined with magnesium or some other mineral. They are deposited on the hair and then fused into the hair with heat.

I believe that the heavy protein I use does not permanently rebuild the structure, but temporarily mimics the healthy structure of the hair. Its effect is temporary, since the treatment is performed every six weeks. If the effect were permanent, the treatment would not need to be repeated at such regular intervals. Furthermore, if the effect were permanent, re-applications would be required to act only on new growth, and the directions would tell you to place the product only at the roots of the hair. Since the product information does not say this, but recommends that the product be placed on the entire length of the hair every time you apply it, it must not be permanent. It is temporary.

The heavy protein product mimics the healthy structure of the hair, but does not actually re-create the hair structure. According to the bulk of the information available today on hair science, it is not possible to repair or rebuild a hair shaft or strand once that hair shaft or strand has been damaged. Damage to the hair is permanent.

Hair is damaged because we handle and style it, and because it ages. Everything wears out over time, including hair. By using a heavy protein treatment, we are trying to extend the length of time a strand of hair remains undamaged-looking by protecting the scale structure of the hair. The rebuilding action of the heavy protein product is purely cosmetic, or temporary.

The two main components of the protein product that I use are modified protein and magnesium. As I mentioned before, magnesium coats the hair. This can help to attract and hold the protein components of a product on the hair, but the coating action can also inhibit the proper processing of permanents, hair coloring and relaxers by blocking their chemistry from reaching the hair. Therefore, always perform a hard-core protein treatment after, and not before, any of the above-mentioned chemical processes.

Modern products designed for dry hair have large molecules that contain positive electrical charges. Hair strands carry a small negative charge, so the positively charged molecules cling to the hairs. The large molecules collect on the edges of the damaged scales of the cuticle, helping to smooth over and fill in the breaks and cracks. The smoothed hair cuticle reflects light better. As a result, the hair tends to become shinier. The smoothed cuticle is less likely to catch on other hairs and become tangled, so the hair becomes more manageable.

Finally, because of the drying effects of the heavy protein, I strongly recommend that the hair be deeply moisturized after a heavy protein treatment.

I have mentioned that mineral-heavy water, especially water heavy in magnesium, may not be great for your hair. Therefore, the recommendation here of a heavy protein product that may contain magnesium might seem like a glaring inconsistency. It is true that in general, magnesium deposited on the hair from hard water is known to create dryness and dullness. However, when you understand your goal and your products and their impact on your hair, you can incorporate a magnesium-heavy product into your routine for the benefit of your hair. You are looking at the big picture, the results you wish to attain in the long run. This is where the idea of having a model for your hair pays dividends.

Many people do not like heavy protein products. I would strongly suggest that you find a protein product that you do like. In order for the protein in the product to remain on the hair and support the natural hair structure over an extended period of time, the composition of the product must be designed in such a way that the protein is infused into the hair strands. This requires that the produce be applied with the use of heat.

All products can eventually be washed out of the hair. When looking for a heavy protein product, you want to find one that does not wash out during your next wash, or within a few days or a week of its use.

To ensure that your results are positive, here are some steps you can follow to have an optimum heavy protein treatment experience. Before you start, please remove all the product build-up from your hair. A clarifying shampoo can help, or you can dissolve one-quarter cup of apple cider vinegar into a quart of warm water and rinse it through the hair. I like to use a wide-mouth bowl of water with apple cider vinegar. First, I detangle my hair with my fingers and loosely braid it. Then I place the top of my head in the bowl and swish my hair around inside the bowl for a few minutes to lift the product.

Heavy Protein Usage Routine:

1. Using your fingers, detangle your hair as completely as possible. Do not leave any major tangles in the hair.

2. Section your hair. Keep it tangle-free by putting the sections into twists or loose braids. Have six to ten sections at most.

3. Heavy protein must be applied on clean hair. Wash the sectioned hair. Dilute one to two caps of shampoo in two to three cups of warm water, so the shampoo doesn't get concentrated in one spot of your hair. This way, you use less shampoo and you can rinse it out more quickly. Rinse the shampoo from your hair.

4. Apply the heavy protein product to your hair. I loosen one braid at a time and pour a capful of the protein product onto the loosened section. Then I braid the section back very loosely, move it out of the way and go on to the next section.

5. After the product has been applied to each section, secure all your hair so that it does not move. I tie my braids up together on the top of my head with a nylon stocking.

6. Sit under a dryer until the product becomes hard.

7. Carefully rinse the product from your hair, without moving the hair. YOUR HAIR WILL BREAK if you are rough, or if

you comb it out at this point. Be gentle! I place my head under the sink and rinse until the product is completely out of my hair. This can take from ten to fifteen minutes. Usually, I do not loosen my hair even when the product has been rinsed out. (Not all heavy protein treatments become hard. Follow the directions of your product for best results.)

8. After the treatment, your hair may be very, very dry. YOU MUST DEEP CONDITION YOUR HAIR AFTER THE TREATMENT. Mix a deep moisturizing conditioner, perhaps one containing cholesterol, or any conditioner of your choice—it should be thick and rich—with olive oil, almond oil, castor oil, wheat germ oil and/or safflower oil. I would suggest for every one fourth cup of conditioner that you add one tablespoon of oil.

9. Unloosen one braid at a time. Mix the oil/conditioner mixture into your loosened hair with your hands. Do not comb the hair at this point.

10. Work the conditioner into every section of hair that you just unbraided. Braid the same section again. Continue with this process until you have placed conditioner throughout your head. Let it sit for five minutes to one hour. I think five to ten minutes is good.

11. Unloosen one braid at a time. Comb the hair out section by section with the conditioner still in it until the hair is completely detangled. Go to the next braid.

12. After each braid has been combed and detangled, twist it or loosely braid it again and move it out of the way. That is why you don't want to have too many braids, not more than ten.

13. Rinse each section. Move each rinsed section out of the way. You can tie the rinsed section up with an old knee-high nylon, adding sections as they are rinsed and detangled, or you can just twist or braid the hair loosely again.

14. Style as usual.

If you don't deep condition after the protein treatment, and if you don't handle your hair very carefully, you could break the hair. Your hair is at its most vulnerable during and immediately after a heavy protein treatment. Once you get the oily conditioner mix in, you should be ready to handle your hair the way you are used to—gently!

Minimize handling of your hair after the deep protein treatment. Just deep condition it and rinse well. Have your towels and clothing ready so that once you have removed the product from your hair, you can perform your normal hair routine. You don't want to walk around the house trying to find a towel with water dripping into your eyes and on the floor. Wait six to eight weeks before applying this treatment again.

Deep Conditioning

Deep conditioning is another way to protect your hair. Assuming that you wash your hair once a week, you should use deep conditioning every time. Deep conditioning entails using a thicker conditioner that is left in the hair for a period of time, anywhere from five minutes to an hour. A deep conditioning treatment can contain protein. Since some people's hair does not do well with protein, I would suggest that you select a deep conditioner that does not contain protein. If you determine that protein works well for your hair, then you can use an additional conditioning product that contains protein. For some people, it may be best to use the protein treatment before the moisturizing deep conditioning treatment. For some, it may be best to use the conditioning treatment first. For others, it may be best to only use the protein treatment or to only use the moisturizing treatment. As I have mentioned throughout, it really is up to you to determine what works best for you. Sometimes trial and error is the only way to make this determination. The more knowledge and understanding you have, the more productive and the shorter that trial and error period is likely to be.

You can use thick store-bought conditioners that indicate on their packaging that they moisturize the hair. You can also use oils infused with herbs to condition your hair. I prefer to use conditioner that I buy from the store, and then use the oils as leave-ins after I have conditioned my hair. Please rinse the conditioner out of your hair before applying a leave-in product.

Leave-In Products

After conditioning my hair, I like to add a leave-in. "Leave-in" is a term for a product that you place in your hair, but you don't rinse it out. It is usually the product that you apply just before you style your hair. I like to create or mix my own leave-in products. Here are some of the components you can use to make your own leave-in:

Strengthener

- Leave-in products containing panthenol
- MSM liquid vitamins taken internally. MSM stands for methyl sulfonyl methane. Raw vegan foods contain high levels of naturally occurring MSM. It is said that MSM works by contributing sulfur for keratin production, which is required for healthy hair.

Conditioner

- Inexpensive conditioner of your choice
- Aloe vera gel from a natural source and not heavily processed or diluted

Moisturizer

- Water
- Vegetable glycerin
- Aloe vera gel

Lubricant

- Vegetable glycerin
- Vegetable oil (olive, castor, almond, sesame, coconut)

Stimulant

⟲ Essential oil of peppermint (1-3 drops)
⟲ Essential oil of tea tree (1-3 drops)

The bulk of my mixture is conditioner and water. I add about one-half cup of one of the other components and place the mixture in a spray bottle. I use the essential oils as indicated, only drops at a time. They are potent and should be respected. Do not pour great quantities of essential oils into your products.

Once I place the leave-in on my hair, if I am wearing a natural style, I like to seal it with a heavier product, which I simply place on top of the leave-in. The heavier products I use may be hair lotions, such as curl activators, or butters, such as mango, aloe, shea, avocado, cocoa or coconut oil. I might use one of these butters by itself, or melt and mix it with some other oil in which I am interested at the time.

To seal my hair, I have also used un-petroleum jelly over the leave-in. Un-petroleum jelly is a product with a petroleum-jelly-like texture, but is made from vegetable products as opposed to petroleum products. My favorite, though, is petroleum jelly. Many people consider petroleum jelly a terrible product for the hair and skin. However, it works for me, so I use it.

Handling While Styling

The final component of the protection step is the handling of the hair.

Styling Methods

There are several ways to style hair. The focus of the styling hints in this book is to help you to retain the length of your hair.

Baggie Method

Simply use a plastic sandwich bag to cover the hair once it has been moisturized and sealed. You can secure the bag over your pony-tail, braids, twists or puffs.

Scarf Method

Cover your hair with a satin or silk scarf to maintain your style and protect the hair. Underneath the scarf, your hair may be straightened and loose or styled in braids or twists, or in a braid-out or twist-out style. Braid-out and twist-out styles are created by braiding or twisting the hair and then loosening it and finger-combing it. Finger-combing the hair, or just leaving it be without even running your fingers through it, helps to maintain the pattern left by the braids and twists after they have been removed.

Extensions Method

You can protect your hair by using hair pieces. The extensions can be in the form of sewn-in weaves, falls, wigs, half-wigs or phony ponytails. These extensions can work just as well as, if not better than, the baggie or scarf method to protect your hair, as long as you maintain the good care of your natural hair underneath the extensions. These styles are the ultimate low-manipulation styles.

Low-Manipulation Method

Another way to protect your hair is not to comb or brush it harshly at all throughout the day. I prefer to comb and detangle my hair only on wash day, but this may not work for everyone. Just keep in mind that you really don't want to be styling, parting, combing or brushing your hair throughout the day. Low manipulation will help protect your hair. Once again, this method is something that you will need to determine how to employ for yourself.

Heat Usage Methods

Lastly, minimize the use of heat and styling tools to protect your hair. Using a curling iron, blow dryer or pressing comb on your hair every day is a sure way to damage the ends. Once the ends are damaged, they may need to be trimmed or cut. This causes you to lose valuable growth. When you retain less of your growth, you have shorter-looking hair.

Find styles that look good without needing a lot of heat. Even cutting back on your use of heat from once a week to only twice a month can make a big difference. I like to use heat in my hair as a treat. I tend to use heat about two times a year. For me, this is not a sacrifice, because I enjoy wearing my natural hair. Again, you will have to determine what works best for you and fits into your lifestyle. Roller setting is an ideal method for minimizing the use of heat. An excellent resource is a DVD entitled, "The Healthy Textures Guide to Roller Setting," with host Gennifer Miller.

How Does the Grow It Way of Protecting Help to Preserve the Structure of the Hair Shaft?

Wearing hair coverings or hair products shields the hair and prevents it from touching anything except itself. The coverings and products form a barrier between your hair and everything else.

In the daytime, the barrier protects your hair from wind, air, ultra-violet rays from the sun, minerals, pollution and clothing. At night, you can cover and protect your hair with scarves, plastic caps, plastic bags, weaves, extensions, wigs and hairstyles that are pulled off and away from clothing. You can also use sealants such as olive, almond, coconut and castor oils, and lotions, creams, petroleum jelly and un-petroleum jelly.

Another way to protect your hair is by the use of a water filter in the shower or tub. Water filters block and minimize the amounts of chlorine and minerals that can be deposited in your hair through showers, baths and general contact with tap water.

Now let us move to Step 6, which focuses on growing your hair.

CHAPTER 14

Step 6
All About Growing

Growing healthy hair to lengths that you have never attained before requires that you shift your thinking. Once you shift your thinking, you must then shift your actions. Both these changes together are required for you to maximize and leverage the growth that you receive.

Shift Your Thinking to Retain Longer Hair

Your actions are what you do or do not do to your hair. I know that this sounds obvious, but it is the obvious, along with all its subtleties, that is often overlooked. Just as the "b" in the words "obvious" and "subtleties" is silent or hidden, the obvious can be hidden and overlooked by the uninitiated, untrained eye. Therefore, let me dig into the obvious, pull out the "B's" and shed some light on them for you.

Beliefs

The first "B" is belief. It is important to believe that what you are trying to do is achievable. If you do not really believe that you can grow your hair to longer lengths, you will sabotage your potential progress and your tangible, real progress. If you do not believe that

81

you can reach your goals, you are likely to quit and give up within weeks, if not days, of starting your growing process. If you don't think you can reach your goals, you are likely to trim or cut away any progress that you have made.

The best way to saturate your mind with new belief is to interact with others who have successfully taken the journey that you wish to take. You can do this easily and with little risk by finding a hair care board or a set of online photo albums that allow the users to share photos and ideas. You can choose to ask questions or simply view the information that is posted on these boards. Looking through other peoples' albums can help you see some of the mistakes they have made as well as their successes, and can give you tips about their processes.

Seeing really is believing. Looking at photographs, especially genuine and authentic progress photographs of someone's hair over time, is a great way to stoke your belief that what you want to do is do-able. Even incremental success, such as getting shine on hair that was once dull, or obtaining a half-inch of growth where there was breakage, can be motivating and empowering. These are just a few ways to get your "belief muscle" strengthened and motivated. Even if your belief is only as small as a mustard seed—and they are tiny!—it will be enough to get you solidly on track. Without belief, it is most difficult to stay the course.

Boundaries

The next "B" is boundaries. I think of boundaries in two ways. The first way I think of boundaries is as the limitations that we unnecessarily place upon ourselves. You never know what you can do if you don't try. Leave the limitations and great expectations behind you. Yes, expectations can be limiting, too. If your expectations don't fit your situation, you can use them to say that you can't reach a goal. For example, you might expect your hair to improve in one month's time. This sounds like a relatively innocuous or harmless expectation, but if I had had such an expectation, it would have been detrimental to my progress and success. My hair does not improve on a month-to-month basis. I have seen many women who have beautiful results after taking better care of their hair for thirty days, but if I had kept this expectation for myself, I would have given up on my hair journey as soon as I found any dry, brittle, broken ends. For me, the expectation of monthly improvement would have been a limitation. You really just have to be open.

The second way I think of crossing boundaries is in the idea of "leaps and bounds." When you are on track, you can take leaps and bounds forward in the progress of your hair. Simply stepping out in faith and trying something new with your hair can cause your confidence to take off in leaps and bounds. When you are confident, it is more difficult for someone's insensitive or intentionally unkind comment to hit its mark. When you take a leap of faith, you can move past many boundaries, especially the boundaries in your own mind. Taking a leap of faith fortifies you so that you can also move past the boundaries other people may throw in your path in the form of negative or ignorant comments. To respond to such comments with anger or hurt, internalizing what people have said or done and allowing it to bother you, is an indicator that you need to leap with faith back onto the path. It is a sign that you have given your power away to those people. Don't do it!

Do not waste precious life energy or time on the limitations and expectations of others, or your own. Focus solely upon yourself and your hair. Your energy and attention will be so much better spent, and it will reap dividends for you and your hair.

Basics

The next "B" that you need is a basic, stabilized hair routine, regimen or process. This means that you need to find some basic products that work for you. "Products that work" does not mean products that give you two inches of growth in three days. A product that works is a product, process or routine that you have implemented which does not damage or harm your hair. No, your hair may not be flourishing, but it is not breaking, either.

Many people believe that they do not have a hair routine or regimen. Everyone has a routine. A routine is whatever you are doing or using today. If you wash your hair every three weeks with dish soap, that is your routine. If you use a series of five different shampoos over five days, that is your routine.

If you are one of those people who use mountains of products, I would suggest that you simplify your routine. Eliminate some of the products and try to get down to a shampoo or cleanser and a conditioner that you like.

Once you have simplified your routine, take a minute to write down whatever you do to your hair. It takes less time to write the information down in an inexpensive little notebook than to rack your brain later, trying to remember what you did to your hair last time. Hair is funny. You never know what may give you a wonderful result. If you get in the habit of writing down what you do to your hair, then when one of those pleasant surprises hits you, you can go back through your notes, find what may have caused your little miracle and repeat it with confidence.

Once you have your basic routine, you have an idea of what is holding your hair steady. If you want to add different products or processes, you will be able to see quickly what may or may not be working for you.

Baseline

The next "B" is the baseline. Baseline refers to the acknowledgement and documentation of your starting point. This starting point becomes your base, against which you will measure and compare all progress and setbacks. You can create a baseline with photographs and notes.

I would strongly suggest that you baseline your progress with photos. Even though it may be painful and uncomfortable for you to look at your hair, take a photograph of your loosened hair from the back, front, top, and the left and right sides. Print these photos if you can, even if you keep an online journal. There is something about a tangible photograph that an online photograph can't match. Keep these photographs in a safe, accessible place so that you can look at them freely whenever you want.

Remember, even if you have been under the care of a beautician or hairstylist for many years, the state of your hair is solely your responsibility. If you blame your hairstylist for the poor condition of your hair or for your lack of hair, you have entirely missed the point of this book. You are the caretaker of your hair. Do not blame someone else for your inability to stand up for your hair, or for not choosing to do what is best and right for your hair. Do not blame yourself, either. Simply accept where you are and vow to take matters into your own hands, to do a better job from today forward.

Blinders

The next "B" is blinders. Many people believe that vision and hearing are purely physiological. They think that these senses are nothing but physical components of the human body. They are not! Sight and hearing are possible in the human experience not only because of the properly working physical components in the body, such as our eyes, nerves and eardrums, but because of properly working physical and psychological processes in our minds and brains.

Unfortunately, people in our world have experienced accidents and traumas. Even if their eyes and/or ears have sustained no physical damage, or the damage has healed, their brains or minds have sustained some internal injury that has adversely affected their vision or hearing. The result is that even with intact and seemingly well-functioning eyes and ears, they are unable to hear or see. Their experiences have created blinders around their ability to perceive the world around them.

You may ask, what does this have to do with hair? The point is that in the case of your hair, your eyes can deceive you. Dealing with your hair is highly personal and emotional. Emotions partly make up your state of mind. Your state of mind influences your perception— how you see your world at any moment. Technically, perception is not reality, but it definitely is *your* reality.

When you loosen your hair and get it blown dry, flat-ironed or straightened, and then you come home and look in the mirror, it is easy to be disappointed by what you see. Here, again, are those boundaries in the form of limitations and expectations. It is so easy to look at your hair and say, "It didn't grow. It didn't get longer." This is, of course, a residue of your old thinking, your old belief system. Do you remember that you have to change your thinking in order to grow your hair to new lengths? This requires more than will power and positive thinking. It requires action. Take a picture! Take a picture!

I cannot tell you the number of times in my hair journey that I looked at my hair in the mirror and believed that I had made no progress. Even when I didn't think it would make any difference, I still took pictures. Taking those pictures made an incredible difference for me, as well as for my hair. Therefore, I truly believe that it is critical to document your hair journey with photographs. It will save you from cutting your hair during those times of utter disappointment, and will help you see with clearer vision where you really are and what progress you have made.

Sometimes, days or even weeks may need to pass before you can get into a good state of mind in which your vision is not clouded by stress, family or financial issues or personal problems. Contrary to what you may think, clear vision does not make the situation seem rosier than it is. Clear vision is razor-sharp, and can be breathtaking in its accuracy. Get it, cultivate it and use it!

If you can, it is ideal to document what products you are using, how you are using them and the frequency with which you are using them. Who knows, applying conditioner to your hair before you wash it as opposed to after you wash it could make a big difference for you. You won't know that unless you write down what you do, how you do it and the result you get from doing it.

Break Points

The last "B" is break points. The point at which your hair always breaks is the point at which you may need to change your routine. This sounds glaringly obvious, but it is hard to see and realize. It is the hardest point to get past.

Let's look at this in more detail. Think back to the longest your hair has ever grown. Even if your hair is still at this length, if it doesn't grow any longer this is likely to be your break point. Another way to look at this is to ask, "How long does my hair get with minimum or no effort on my part?" This length is considered your break point.

To get past this point, I suggest that you take three steps. Every step requires that you gain knowledge and information, and use it. It is that simple. Remember, it is often the obvious that eludes us.

1. Identify the break point. Be conscious. Observe.

2. Do not fear the break point and thus be prevented from doing anything.

3. Get ready for it. Take some action!

We have already talked about how to identify the break point. Knowledge is a great opponent of fear. Fear can sometimes lock you in place, which may be why we continue to perform the same processes as we always do at our break point. Knowledge can fortify you and help you get past being fearful. Bathe yourself in knowledge. Let knowledge be your shield. Use it to get ready to move past your break point and reach new, longer lengths.

In general, hair may have different needs at different lengths. Here are some observations that I have made, based upon my experience.

Fastest Growth Point: Shoulder Length

Hair grows most quickly from a shaved head to a small Afro, from Afro to puff, from one inch long to the neck, from the ears to neck and from the ears to the shoulder. Shoulder length is not only one of the fastest growth points, but it is also one of the most notorious break points. Until your hair has reached shoulder length, wearing puffs, twists and braids can be helpful in maintaining and supporting the growth of your hair. Usually, in these styles, the ends of the hair are out, unprotected and exposed to the air. For the most part, the lack of protection of the ends of the hair in these styles does not affect the health of the hair. Often, the hair has been newly cut or trimmed, and the strand is young and has not had a lot of time to age and wear. However, once the hair hits shoulder length, these styles can have a negative impact on the retention of its growth.

Once your hair reaches shoulder length, look over your routine to determine whether you should modify it. In most cases, I believe that you should modify your routine at this stage. Because your hair has reached your shoulders, the frail and vulnerable ends can be caught under a heavy book bag or purse strap, entwined in the threads of your clothing or smashed between your head and whatever support you are using for your head, neck and back. To prevent this, during the day you can pin your ends up or put them in a baggie covered by a hat or scarf, or you can wear a phony ponytail over them. You have an entire menu of protective styles from which to use. Choose a couple and determine which ones work best for you.

To fortify the ends of your hair at night, place oil on them. If you and your style can support it, place a little cream or a heavier oil over the first oil. If your hair does not like oil, spray your ends with water or a water-based concoction and tuck the ends up overnight.

Most Common Break Points: after Shoulder Length, before Waist Length

The most common points of breakage are from shoulder length to just under the armpit, from armpit length to mid-back, and from mid-back to the bra strap. Most women fall off the track of their hair-growing process at the point between the shoulder blades and bra strap. This is a large area to cover.

Because each person is different, you are going to have to use knowledge, your photos, your entire routine and regimen to determine what you need to do at this juncture. You may discover that at your newer length, you have discovered a new break point. Apply the break point formula: identify it, don't fear it and get ready for it. Be open to trying different styling options, and to providing more care and attention to the ends.

Slowest Growth Points: from Bra-Strap to Waist Length, from Waist to Hip Length

Based upon what I have observed, from bra strap to waist and from waist to hip are the slowest points of growth. The interesting part is that some of your hair will grow quickly to these lengths, but getting the bulk of your hair even and thick at these lengths takes lots of time and care. Therefore, these are the slowest growth points to reach.

It is at these lengths where the Goal Point method can be the most useful. I use this method at such points to thicken up the ends of my hair. The Goal Point method is described in detail in a later section.

When small amounts of hair reach these points, I acknowledge that this is my newest goal length, and I go into action. I verify that my newer Goal Point length is no more than two to four inches longer than the rest of my hair. If you have too much distance between your longest hairs and the bulk of your hair, you may feel that it is taking too long for the bulk of the hair to catch up with those few long hairs. This may cause you to be more likely to cut or trim the ends back. Then you will feel discouraged by what you may perceive as your lack of progress. If you keep the distance between the bulk of your hair and the longest ends shorter, you will have less time to wait before you see the bulk catch up to the longer hair. This shorter waiting time may cause you to be more likely to stick to your regimen and your process, and attain that longer length.

If the distance between the bulk and the ends is more than two to four inches, you can always trim the ends back a little until the distance is no more than recommended. Then keep your hair trimmed at the newer length, and nurture it.

Picture taking is especially important at two points: when you are growing the hair to your waist and to your hips. These are the two stages at which I thought my hair had stopped gaining length. However, because I was able to look at my pictures, I realized that the sides had indeed grown longer, or that the middle had become thicker and fuller. These things may not have had an impact on extending the length of the bulk of my hair, but they certainly had an impact on my state of mind.

At those stages, because I believed that my hair had stopped gaining length, I was tempted to cut it as much as a couple of inches, to thicken it at what I thought was my permanent, or terminal, length. That would have been a grave error. Because I had the pictures, I was able to retain the "just maybe" attitude in my mind and keep going on faith.

The common element snaking its way through all these break points is that as the hair gets longer, it gets older. The hair mirrors your life: the older it is, the more fragile it is likely to be. You can strengthen your hair with the products you use, the food you eat and whatever you put into your body. Still, simply because the hair is older, it is more frequently exposed to situations of breakage. Even though you may be handling your hair carefully and treating it like silk or satin, the mere fact that it is older makes it prone to breakage.

I guess older hair can be compared with a senior citizen who is in supreme health. Even if you are a person who has arrived at your twilight years in pristine health, there are certain things your body just won't allow you to do anymore. Understanding this is not placing a limitation on yourself—it is using common sense.

Constantly pulling and stretching older, longer hair may eventually break it. Don't test it. Yes, your hair will become stronger and healthier as your arsenal of knowledge improves. However, always keep the awareness in the back of your mind that the longer your hair is, the older it is likely to be. Treat your longer hair like the senior citizen it is. Honor it and continue to handle it gently. Keep in mind that every time you handle your hair, you are presented with a new opportunity either to venerate and honor it by handling it carefully and consciously, or to damage it further, drawing it back into the cycle of setbacks and breakage.

Shift Your Actions to Retain Longer Hair

Condition of the Hair Ends

Are full ends—ends that are thick and even—created or grown? For those rare individuals whose hair all grows to the same length at the same time, full ends are grown. For others, mere mortals, full hair ends can be created. That is great news!

The creation of full ends is not product-dependent, but thought- and action-dependent. Ideally, ends look fuller when the following is apparent:

- the bulk of the hair is all at the same length
- the ends are evenly trimmed
- the hair is free from split ends
- the ends are not broken or damaged
- the ends are not brittle and dry, and do not have a dull gray cast or color

The Goal Point method is one way to get your ends to the same length. A trusted friend or professional can help you trim your ends so that they are all at the same length. Trims can also help with the eradication of visible split ends. Protecting your hair ends can help them stay soft, smooth and moisturized.

If the very bottom of your hair is thinner than the bulk of the hair, or if you can see through the ends more than through the rest of your hair, you have thin ends. "Thin ends" is a relative term. You should not compare the thickness of your hair to another person's. If your hair is the same thickness from root to tip, yet it is thinner than your friend's hair, this does not necessarily mean that you have thin ends. Your hair is simply finer or thinner overall than someone else's. On the other hand, if the hair on your head has more thickness or fullness near the roots than it does as you move down the hair shaft, you have thin, or thinner, ends.

In Afro-textured natural hair, thin ends can mean either that your hair is breaking or that it is growing. If you see that your hair has thin ends, how do you tell if this is good or bad? First, put the scissors down and hold off with the trim until you make a decision.

If you can, straighten your hair or stretch it. Since you are looking at the ends, you don't want to pull and stretch only a section at a time. It is best to straighten or stretch out all of your hair at once. Now take a good, clear photograph of the back of your head, to measure the length. Then continue performing your routine or regimen for at least a month, four weeks at a minimum. At the end of this period, straighten your hair again and take another photograph.

The critically important first photograph is your baseline measurement. After the four weeks have passed, look at the second photo. If your hair is shorter than or the same length as it was before and your ends are thin, it is likely that your hair is breaking. If your hair is longer than the last time you measured it, but it is see-through or a bit thinner at the very ends, it is most likely growing to longer lengths.

If your hair is breaking, you need to stabilize it. Try to identify the reason your hair is breaking. There are several possible causes. Use your photographs and notes of your products, routine and results to help identify or eliminate potential culprits or problems. If your hair has grown in length but it has thin ends, determine whether you want to retain the gain in length or cut it. If you decide you want to retain that gain, use the Goal Point method detailed directly below.

Goal Point Method: How to Reach Newer, Longer Lengths

Accepting Transition

Uneven hair is hair that is shaped like a V or a Y at the bottom, or hair in which the line of the ends looks jagged. One of the hardest steps to take is to get past the idea that uneven hair is necessarily unhealthy hair. It is not. In many situations, uneven hair only seems to be unhealthy because it is not even and neat. That even and neat-looking result is just that: an end state, or goal, that you are trying to reach. In order to get there, you have to take the appropriate steps. The uneven hair is just hair in a transitional state, not necessarily hair in an unhealthy state.

We all know that before we end up at that final "changed" state, there are steps that must be taken. That's for other people, though, not for us. Right? Wrong! It's for you, too. If you want your hair to look perfectly even at every step and stage of its gain in length, you can accomplish that, but please understand that the speed at which you retain length will be retarded. This is neither wrong nor right. However, if you want to grow your hair as fast as you can and optimize the new length you have received, trimming your hair to keep it even is definitely the wrong way to do it.

It is all a matter of placing things in context. You must expect to have uneven hair at some point in your journey. What you do with it will determine whether your hair does well at this newer length.

Our key assumptions now are that you have a basic routine and you are protecting your ends. If these components are in place, the most likely result is that your hair may be uneven, but it is not damaged. Remember, though, that some split ends are inevitable. No matter how well you treat your hair, you will be likely to get a few.

While you are waiting for the bulk of your hair to drop to the length of the longer hair, you still want to look and feel good about your hair. Try to find styles that do not rely upon evenly trimmed hair for their beauty. Braided, twisted and curly hair styles are all styles that would fit this transitional time.

Use some imagination and experimentation to find a style or several styles that you like to wear. If you do not feel attractive and enjoy the styling options you are using, you are not likely to continue on your growing path. It takes some effort to find the styles you enjoy, but we all know that without effort, your hair will remain at its normal break point length.

When and Why to Use the Goal Point Method

All hair strands do not grow to the same length at the same rate, all at the same time. If you are growing your hair to new lengths, the bulk of the hair will not be the longest hair. Still, theoretically, if one strand of hair can get to a longer length, the rest can, too. Single hair strands and small sections of hair will increase in length first. This method allows you to recognize, nurture, support and protect these lone hair strands until the rest catches up.

How to Use the Goal Point Method

1. Determine the goal point. Your goal point is likely to be the newest length your hair has reached. Lead hairs, or the hairs that have reached a longer length than the rest of your hair, are your indicators.

2. Don't let the lead hairs get more than two to four inches longer than the rest of the hair. The reasons for this are twofold. First, the longer, thinner hair will become too hard to manage, since it is vulnerable and can break. Second, you may become impatient if you have too much distance, or length, between the bulk of your hair and the lead hair.

3. Nurture and protect the lead hair. Keep the lead hair at your goal length. This is the length you want the bulk of the hair to reach. This simply means that you should keep the lead hair trimmed at the point you have designated as your goal length. Don't let that lead hair grow past the goal point length.

4. Once the bulk of the hair reaches the lead hair, trim it even. Trim the bulk of the hair to match the length of the lead hair. Please keep in mind that as the bulk of the hair gets longer, the lead hair may drop in length, too. That is why you should always know exactly where on your body your goal point length is located. The next time you stretch or pull your hair straight, you may find that the lead hair has grown past the

goal point, and the bulk of the hair has either reached the goal point or passed it, too. Once again, pictures are a great tool to use in determining whether the hair is reaching or passing your goal point.

This is how you thicken up your ends to create fuller, thicker-looking hair from root to tip. Thick, full ends at your goal point—in other words, a whole new length—is the wonderful result.

When you use the Goal Point method, you can see which hair, hairs or sections of hair drop in length first. The lead hair may be on the side, in the middle of the back, or in back on the right or left side of your head. This lead hair indicates the next length you may reach, and it shows you how your hair grows. This is your growing pattern. If you know your growing pattern, you can use this knowledge to reach longer lengths and to avoid trimming your hair prematurely.

Trim Conscientiously, Keeping Your Goal in Mind

As part of your overall method of gaining length, trimming hair the right way is one of those painfully obvious steps that is really not so obvious and straightforward when you are dealing with your own tresses, which you have worked so hard to maintain. Instead of agonizing over what you should do, let's look at some options. These can help you determine what is best for you.

Should you trim your hair when it is natural or straightened?

This depends on your preferred styling options. For me, it is not important that my natural hair hang at an even length. The ends of my hair tend to curl and twist and draw up, hiding their true length, anyway.

I do like to wear my hair straightened for special events, though. That is when I like to see full, beautiful, evenly trimmed ends. This trim can be blunt cut, U-shaped or V-shaped. You can have full ends with all these shapes, so it really doesn't matter which one you choose. For me, what matters is that my straightened hair is even and full. Therefore, I prefer to have my hair trimmed when it is straightened.

Because our hair tends to draw up when it is natural, I don't do any kind of trimming or cutting when my hair is in its natural state. One wrong snip can set my progress back for weeks, if not months. On the other hand, if you know that your main style is one that is natural and un-straightened or un-stretched, then by all means, trim your hair this way, in its natural state.

In summary, trim and shape your hair according to the style that is important to you. You just have to determine how you want to wear your hair.

Should you trim your hair when it is braided or twisted, or when it is loosened?

Even if you keep your hair natural and never straighten it, you still need to make a conscious decision about when to trim. Some women trim off split ends while their hair is styled in twists and braids. If you don't mind how your hair is shaped when you unfurl your mane and wear it loosened, then go ahead and trim it while it is braided or twisted.

However, remember that when the hair is braided you cannot see your whole head, and so you run the risk of cutting a section of hair shorter than the rest. If it is possible that you are going to decide later on that you want to wear it loose, you will probably want symmetrical or even-looking hair. Then you may be tempted to "fix" the too-short section by going over your entire head to even it up. By the time you've evened it up, you may look in the mirror and see that you have somehow cut away all your new length. That is a bad realization to have after the fact.

Cutting your hair to re-shape it is not a bad thing to do. Just be conscious, and do your trimming with the realization of what the outcome may be. That way, you will minimize your regrets. You will trim with knowledge and understanding, and will arrive at your length intentionally and not by accident.

Should you trim your hair dry or wet?

This really depends on your type of hair and your personal preference. My hair is still curly when it is wet, and it can be different lengths at different times, depending upon where the water is hitting it or where it is wetter. Therefore, wet hair is too unreliable for me to trim. I prefer to trim my hair dry and straightened.

Some women's hair is super-straight when it is wet. They are able to see clearly what needs to be trimmed. If this were my situation, I would definitely trim it when it was wet. Again, you have to determine what is best for you.

How often should you trim?

If you have reached a length that you really enjoy and you want to keep your hair at that length, I suggest that you trim your hair every six to eight weeks. That's enough time between trims to get a half to one inch of growth. If your hair all grows to the same length at once, this will help it reach the next length evenly with thick, full ends.

I do not trim that often because my hair does not all grow to the same length at the same time. Once I stabilized my routine and began the use of protective styles and processes, I found that I could go for longer periods without my ends getting frayed. I experimented. I started going for six months, twelve months and eighteen months without a trim.

I found that twelve months without a trim was the optimum time frame while I was growing my hair out. Six months didn't give me enough time to get most of the bulk at the newer length. Eighteen months made my expectations too high about the length I thought I'd find at the end of that time, so that when I finally straightened and trimmed my hair after eighteen months, I was disappointed with the result. It was also too long a time frame for my fragile ends to last without breaking.

Once again, you will need to look at your situation and determine what is best for you. There are lots of options. The process is always the same.

How much should you trim?

In determining how much to trim, I always go back to the Goal Point method: I trim my hair where the bulk of the hair has reached the newer, longer length.

There are times when I have reached a new length and the ends of my hair are not as healthy as I would like them to be. Sometimes, I have to cut those ends shorter than I would like. There are also times when my new growth is long and thin and may have some split ends. At these times, I have sometimes retained the length and only trimmed back one-eighth to one-fourth of an inch. It comes down to knowing what your goals are and being conscious of those goals each time you decide to get your hair trimmed.

How Does the Goal Point Method of Growing Help to Preserve the Structure of the Hair Shaft?

The Goal Point method restrains you from cutting away your progress without thinking. Getting your hair into a different, better condition from what you have today and taking it from the length you have today to one that you have never had before requires a paradigm shift, or a shift in your thinking. This shift in thinking has an impact on your actions.

Everyone knows that in order to obtain a new or different result, it is logical to change our actions. But how many of us continue to do the same thing day after day, and then ask why nothing has changed? This is because even though we are logical beings, we need to be able to buy into a new idea or action emotionally before we attach ourselves to the idea and make the change that will help us reach the outcome we desire. We need to be able to feel and believe, and to connect the new action to the belief that it is going to get us to our goal. Logic does not create these connections. Emotions do.

In terms of hair growth, the Goal Point model keeps your goals at the forefront of your mind. It is a reminder that helps you believe and feel that what you wish to achieve is attainable. Perhaps you will think twice before cutting or trimming away your growth, because now, instead of thinking, "Oh, I'll never get there," you think, "Just maybe!"

The Goal Point method of trimming helps us to satisfy our psychological need to see progress. You get to hang onto those healthy strands with a conscious goal in mind. The Goal Point method will not create thick hair where the hair is thin, but it will help you to achieve hair ends that are full and even. This process will get you to longer lengths faster, because you are not cutting away your small gains, the way you would if you were trimming without thinking and without a clear goal in mind.

Psychologically, this method of trimming is much more satisfying. Not only are you gaining length, but also you are able to keep it without your hair becoming or looking unhealthy. Remember, uneven ends are not necessarily unhealthy ends. If you have a solid understanding of this, you'll be less likely to fold because of pressure from your friends and your stylist during your pursuit of longer lengths.

CHAPTER 15

Building Healthier, Longer Hair

The Grow It Process consists of a series of steps to be performed in a specific order on a regular basis, with the sole purpose of helping to preserve the structure of the hair shaft for as long as possible. The more time the hair structure remains in place, intact and undamaged, the more chance you have to reach your longer hair goals.

The implementation of this model will result in longer, healthier hair. If we structure it like a pyramid, with the initial step at the base, this is what we see:

The Grow It Model

Step 6	**Growth**	*Change your thinking*
Step 5	**Protect**	*Shield the hair from everything*
Step 4	**Moisturize**	*Soften the hair structure and make it pliable*
Step 3	**Condition**	*Smooth the cuticles and direct the hair downward*
Step 2	**Cleanse**	*Minimize wear on the hair through decreased manipulation*
Step 1	**Detangle**	*Minimize damage to the hair by reducing the stress placed on it*

Moving from a Vicious Cycle to a Virtuous Cycle

Benefits of a Stabilized Routine

Once your hair is stabilized, you have little or no breakage, no severe detangling issues and/or no shedding (shedding is the loss of an unusually large amount of hair during grooming). You have found what works for you.

If you feel the need to experiment, this is the opportune time to tweak or change your regimen, or to try out new products or processes that interest you. Change only one step or product at a time. Otherwise, it may be too difficult to discern which new product or process worked for you and which did not. One change, if it is done incorrectly, could toss you right back off track and into the vicious cycle again.

Document Your Growth

Take photographs and place them where you can refer to them. Photographs can help you see. They show you what the mind and eyes cannot see. Write down your hair goals, routines, concoctions, and your epiphanies and realizations about your hair. Written information along with the photographs helps you to determine patterns in your hair as well as in your own behavior.

Power Comes from the Attainment of Your Hair Goals

When you attain your hair goals, your success spills over into other areas of your life. You have set goals, created a plan to reach those goals and implemented the plan. Along the way, you have modified the plan to fit your circumstances so that you can better reach your goals. This is goal-setting. It can be applied to any and every facet of your life.

Reaching your hair goals makes you feel good not just because you look good, but because you have accomplished something that is important to you. This is extremely empowering. Take this feeling and the actions you performed to create it, and duplicate it in other areas of your life. Create this feeling of power and accomplishment in your education and training, in your career, with your health, your relationships and your financial situations. Nothing breeds success like success!

Use Your Voice, Literally and Figuratively

Reaching your hair care goals requires that you speak up and determine what is best for you and what is not right for you. Only you can determine which procedures, processes and routines work for you. This requires trial and error. You have to take action and think for yourself. No one can and no one should give you the deciding answers. People can shout many answers to you, but ultimately, you have to make the decision. You have to find the right answer. It's all on you!

All hair stylists are not bad. They are professionals who provide a service. As with any professional, you must guide them in order to obtain maximum satisfaction from their services. You need to be able to communicate what you want clearly. If you are not getting what you want, you need to have enough courage and respect for yourself to get up and leave. You have to know definitively what you need and want before you sit in that stylist's chair. Otherwise, you will often be sorely disappointed.

Don't bad-mouth hair care specialists, generalize and make blanket statements about them. There are good ones and bad ones. Learn to bring out the best in people and situations, so that they are beneficial for you and others.

The Grow It Process in Review

Correct implementation of the Grow It Process results in longer life for the scale structure of the individual strands of hair. This means that each hair has a longer period of time to grow before it fractures and splits.

When you use the Grow It Process, you can minimize the damage done to your hair and better preserve your hair over time. This is likely to result in hair with fewer split ends. Hair that is healthy with minimum damage is stronger and less likely to break. Hair that is not breaking has a greater potential to reach longer lengths in a healthier state than hair that keeps breaking.

Step 1: Detangling with the Fingers

Mechanical implements, such as brushes and combs, can strip the scale structure of your individual hair strands, leaving the interior components of the hair exposed and thus damaging the hair. Use your fingers to detangle your hair. This reduces the possibility of stripping the hair's scale structure.

Step 2: Cleansing

Proper cleansing methods help keep the hair free of excessive tangles and mineral build-up, which can block treatments, dry the hair and increase product build-up. Braiding the hair before cleansing decreases manipulation, protects the scale structure and minimizes the need for the use of mechanical implements, such as brushes and combs. A clarifying cleansing once a month helps to remove product build-up.

Step 3: Conditioning

When hair is wet, it is fragile but also flexible. Natural Afro-textured hair is more vulnerable to damage when it is combed and brushed while dry, because it is less pliable and flexible when it is dry.

Therefore, the lesser of the two "evils" is to comb it when it is wet and lubricated. The best time to do this is at the conditioning stage.

Step 4: Moisturizing

When the hair is kept moist, the scales do not get hard. Moisture helps to preserve the structure by keeping the hair pliable and flexible. This prevents the hair from getting too dry and brittle, which makes it prone to breakage.

Step 5: Protecting the Hair

Minimize exposing your hair to environmental hazards: the rays of the sun, wind and oxidizing chemicals such as chlorine and mineral-heavy hard water. You can cover and protect your hair inexpensively.

As a pricier alternative, you can purchase a water filter for the bathtub and/or shower. Depending upon where it is placed, a water filter can drastically reduce the amounts of chlorine and minerals in your bath and shower water. The reduction of minerals in the water results in the softening of hard water. When fewer minerals are deposited in your hair, the amount of product build-up is reduced. Smaller amounts of minerals in your water mean that smaller amounts of product resins are attracted to and built up on the hair.

Step 6: Growing the Hair

The Grow It Process tries to minimize damage to the scale structure of the hair by implementing techniques that preserve the integrity of the hair structure. Inevitably, hair wears out from age and general wear and tear. The goal is to create a grooming process that will help to prolong the life of the scale, or cuticle, structure of your hair.

The longer the scale structure is in place, the more likely it is that your hair will appear healthy. The longer your hair can remain healthy, the longer the time frame you have to retain growth. The more growth you retain, the better the possibility that you can reach new, longer lengths. Grow it!

References

Frangie, Catherine M. *Milady's Standard Cosmetology*, Thomson Delmar Learning, USA. 2008

Gray, John. *The World of Hair: A Scientific Companion*. From D and G Hair Care Research Center, New York. 1997

Hallal, John. *Milady's Hair-Care Product and Ingredients Dictionary*. Thompson Delmar Learning, Canada. 2004

Hampton, Aubrey. *Natural Organic Hair and Skin Care: Including A to Z Guide to Natural and Synthetic Chemicals in Cosmetics*, 1st Edition. Organica Press, Florida. 1987

Hampton, Aubrey. *What's in Your Cosmetics? A Complete Consumer's Guide to Natural and Synthetic Ingredients*. Odonian Press, Arizona. 1995

Michalun, Natalie and Michalun, Varinia, *Skin Care and Cosmetic Ingredients Dictionary (Milady's Skin Care and Cosmetics Ingredients Dictionary)*. Milady Publishing Company, New York. 1994

Smeh, Nikolaus J. *Creating Your Own Cosmetics—Naturally: The Alternative to Today's Harmful Cosmetic Products*. Alliance Publishing Company, Virginia. 1995

Cosmetic Mall (www.cosmeticmall.com)

Hair Coloring Tips (www.haircoloringtips.com)

Malibu Wellness (www.mailibuwellness.com)

Ask a Scientist (http://www.newton.dep.anl.gov/askasci/gen99/gen99504.htm)

Wise Geek (wisegeek.com)

CPSIA information can be obtained at www.ICGtesting.com
Printed in the USA
LVOW061756150312

273255LV00005B/150/P